# Dana Carpender's Carbohydrate Gram Counter

Completely Revised and Updated

# Dana Carpender's Carbohydrate Gram Counter

## Completely Revised and Updated

### Usable Carbs, Protein, and Calories—
### Plus Tips on Eating Low-Carb!

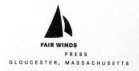

**FAIR WINDS**
PRESS
GLOUCESTER, MASSACHUSETTS

First published in the USA in 2004 by
Fair Winds Press
33 Commercial Street
Gloucester, MA 01930

08 07 06          4 5

ISBN - 13: 978-1-59233-144-4
ISBN - 10: 1-59233-144-0

Library of Congress Cataloging-in-Publication Data available

Original book design by Leslie Haimes and *tabula rasa*
Book design and production by Yee Design

Printed and bound in Canada

*Special thanks to Helena Schaar for compiling the data in this book. She is a
licensed, registered health care professional, college faculty member, and medical
writer with over thirty published articles and books, and fifteen years of experience.
Helena is a lifelong devotee of health and fitness, including calorie counting, good
nutrition, and plenty of exercise.*

**Note:**
*The data is accurate at the time of publication. However, food manufacturers may
change their ingredients at any time without notice.*

# Contents

# Introduction

Hello, low-carb dieter! Whether you're new to the low-carb lifestyle, or have been doing this for a while, I hope you'll find this book a useful tool for achieving weight loss, abundant energy, and robust good health.

I've written a lot of words about the low-carbohydrate lifestyle in the past few years, and I won't try to repeat them all here. But I would like to offer the condensed version, as it were—what I feel are the most vital tips for low-carb success.

## Basic Stuff

- First, and perhaps most important, be clear on this: Whatever you do to lose weight is what you must do for the rest of your life to keep it off. And if carbs are a health problem for you now, they will continue to be a health problem for you until the day you die. Get it through your head that there is no finish line.

- Because you're in this for life, don't focus on losing your weight as quickly as possible. Instead, work on making low-carbing the enjoyable lifestyle it can be, while still achieving your goals. In particular, do not decide that if low carb is good, no carb is better, and cut out everything but eggs, meat, and cheese. You can't eat that way forever, and you know it. You need to incorporate the widest variety of low-carb foods you can, to add flavor and interest, not to mention vitamins, minerals, and fiber.

- It's important to know about "impact carbs," "usable carbs," "net carbs," or "effective carbs." These terms all refer to the grams of carbohydrate that you can actually digest and absorb. What carbohydrates can't you digest or absorb? Fiber! The carbohydrate chains that make up dietary fibers are just too big for the human gut to digest and absorb, which is why we can't live on grass like cows do. Accordingly, you can subtract the grams of fiber from the total grams of carbohydrate to get the number of grams of carbohydrate you actually need to worry about. In this book, we call this number "usable carbs" or "net carbs." This approach dramatically increases the amount of vegetables, fruits, nuts, seeds, and other plant foods you can eat.

- It is my experience that a low-carbohydrate diet is a superb way to overcome genuine obesity and the health problems that come with it—but that it's not particularly useful for achieving that fashionably anorexic look. If you're a size 4 trying to become a size 0, I probably can't help you, and furthermore, I don't want to! It's about health, not about making yourself vanish!

- If you're new to low-carbing, be aware that the first week can be rough. If, like most people, you've been giving your body a little carbohydrate every few hours, your body is used to running on sugar, and probably hasn't been making much use of the enzymes you need to burn fat for fuel. If you burn through your body's stores of sugar before your fat-burning enzyme levels increase, you may "bonk"—feel terribly tired and wrung-out for a day or two. Not everyone goes through this—I didn't—but if it happens to you, know that for most people it lasts no more than a few days. When it's over, you'll be burning fat for fuel, and have more energy than you ever imagined, because you're carrying your supply with you.

- If, along with feeling tired, you feel kind of achy, weak, or crampy, potassium loss—called "hypokalemia"—is likely to be your problem. And if this happens to you, get more potassium right away. Your heart needs potassium to run properly! Don't mess around. The best low-carb source of potassium is avocados; little black ones have 8 grams of usable carb apiece, and

1,200 mg of potassium. Green leafy vegetables are also a good low-carb source of potassium, as are fresh pork, fresh fish, cantaloupe, and almonds. Indeed, it's best to include these things in your diet from Day One.

- You can also take potassium tablets, if you like, but be aware that the doses tend to be low—just 99 mg per tablet, when you need 2,000–3,000 mg of potassium per day. Another way to supplement is to use Morton's Lite Salt, which combines the usual sodium-based salt with potassium-based salt.

  **CAUTION:** If you are on blood pressure medication of any kind, check with your pharmacist or doctor before taking potassium supplements. Some blood-pressure medications work by making your body hang on to potassium, and that makes it possible to get too much, which is as dangerous as too little.

- Potassium imbalance is a temporary problem, caused by your body shifting over from a high-carb diet, which makes you throw off potassium and retain water, to a low-carb diet—which makes you dump all that excess water before your body stops throwing off the potassium. Just eat your good potassium sources, and your body will sort it all out in a week or two.

## Finding YOUR Low-Carb Lifestyle

- There are many approaches to controlling carbohydrates in your diet. If all you've heard about is Atkins and/or *The South Beach Diet*, and you've been unhappy or uncomfortable on these diets, don't give up—do some research, and find the approach that works for your body and your life. To shamelessly plug my own book, in *How I Gave Up My Low Fat Diet and Lost 40 Pounds*, I outline more than a half-a-dozen different approaches to controlling your carbohydrate intake, and therefore your insulin levels. No need for a one-size-fits-all diet.

- Pay attention to your body to learn your "critical carbohydrate level"—the number of grams per day of carbohydrate you must stay below in order to lose weight. For most people this will be between 15 and 60 grams per day. Only time and attention will tell you your critical carbohydrate level.

- You can get an idea of where your critical carbohydrate level is likely to be by finding out how many of the signs of carbohydrate intolerance you have. Here's a list of indicators. How many of them apply to you?

  ☐ I have had a weight problem since I was quite young.

  ☐ I have bad energy slumps, especially in the late afternoon.

  ☐ I get tired and/or shaky when I get hungry.

  ☐ I'm depressed and irritable for no reason.

  ☐ I binge badly or frequently on carbohydrate foods.

  ☐ I carry most of my weight on my abdomen.

  ☐ I have high blood pressure.

  ☐ I have high triglycerides.

  ☐ I have high cholesterol.

  ☐ I have adult onset diabetes.

  ☐ I have heart disease.

  ☐ I have had a female cancer (breast, cervical, ovarian, uterine).

  ☐ I have had a stroke.

  ☐ I am an alcoholic.

  ☐ I have polycystic ovarian syndrome, or the symptoms of it.

  ☐ Obesity runs in my family.

☐ High blood pressure runs in my family.

☐ High triglycerides run in my family.

☐ High cholesterol runs in my family.

☐ Adult onset diabetes runs in my family.

☐ Heart disease runs in my family.

☐ Female cancers run in my family
   (breast, cervical, ovarian, uterine).

☐ Stroke runs in my family.

☐ Alcoholism runs in my family.

☐ Polycystic ovarian syndrome runs in my family.

- If your answer is "yes" to more than three of these, you're likely to be pretty carb-intolerant. The more yes answers, and the more people in your family have these problems, the more intolerant you're likely to be. Keep this in mind when choosing an approach.

- If you have any of the health problems listed above, it is imperative that you be under a doctor's supervision during at least the first few months of going low carb. Blood pressure can come down so quickly that if your medication isn't adjusted you'll get dizzy. Your customary dosage of diabetes medication may suddenly be enough to drop your blood sugar uncomfortably low. If you have trouble with high cholesterol and triglycerides you need a baseline to work from, or you won't know if you've gotten better or worse. Don't be stupid. If your doctor won't cooperate, find one that will, but don't fly blind.

- Most people see an across-the-board improvement in their coronary risk factors—cholesterol, triglycerides, and HDL/LDL ratio—on a low-carb diet, even when eating red meat and high fat dairy foods. However, a minority will see a decrease in triglycerides and an increase in HDL, which is good, but also see a jump in their LDL, which is not so good. If this happens to you, weigh your low-carb diet in favor of fish, poultry, and pork (which is now very lean), use lean cuts when eating beef or lamb, and choose olive oil, nuts, and avocados—sources of monounsaturated fats—over butter, sour cream, and cheese.

## Staying Happy

- In the pursuit of low-carb happiness, especially in the early stages, sit down and brainstorm a list of all of your favorite low-carb foods. What foods do you really love that you've been denying yourself because they were high fat and high calorie? Lobster with butter? Macadamia nuts? Deviled eggs? Brie? Really give this list some thought. Then buy or cook this stuff, and eat it! A great way to stave off feelings of deprivation.

- Buy at least one low-carb cookbook. Shamelessly plugging my own work again, *500 Low-Carb Recipes* is the most popular low-carb cookbook in the US. People tell me they like it because it doesn't call for a lot of weird ingredients, and has a lot of simple recipes that their families like. But there are plenty of other low-carb cookbooks on the market, many of them quite good. The point is, start exploring your kitchen options, instead of letting yourself get locked into fried eggs for breakfast, a bunless burger for lunch, and a plain steak for dinner.

- Make a list of ways to reward yourself that don't involve food. A massage, an hour in a hot bath with a good book, a manicure and pedicure, a phone call to an old friend you haven't talked to in forever—whatever you can think of that will make you feel rewarded, but won't make you fat, sick, and tired. When you've had a hard week, or reached a personal goal, give yourself one of these rewards, instead of carb-y garbage that will only hurt you in the long run.

- When you've lost your first ten or fifteen pounds, buy yourself something wonderful and new to wear—it's a terrific incentive. It's not a bad idea to do this every time you drop another size, if you can afford it, rather than waiting until you've reached your goal weight to buy new clothes. New clothes celebrate and show off your success, and keep you on track.

## About Labels

- Read the labels on everything you put in your mouth. Most people do far more research before buying a car or a DVD player than they do on what they put into their own bodies. "You are what you eat" is literally true. All your body has to make itself from is what you put in your mouth. If you give your body junk, you'll be made out of junk, and you'll feel and look like it. Read the labels even on things you've looked up in this book, or have purchased before—formulas change.

- Having read the labels, choose the products with the lowest carb counts. You can shave untold thousands of grams off of your yearly intake this way. For example, I have seen ham with 1 gram of carbohydrate per serving, and I have seen ham with 6 grams of carbohydrate per serving. That's a 600 percent difference!

- There is no such thing as good sugar! Obviously, sugar, brown sugar, and corn syrup are all bad for you. However, so are the "natural" and "healthy" alternatives like honey, concentrated fruit juice, Sucanat, dried sugar cane juice, malt syrup, rice syrup, turbinado, fructose, dextrose, maltose, or anything else ending in "ose." All of it is sugar, and all of it will cause an insulin release.

- Many alcoholic beverages quote low-carb counts on the labels, and hard liquor, technically speaking, has none. However, alcohol, no matter how low carb, will slow your metabolism dramatically—you'll stop burning fat until your body has metabolized all of the alcohol. This doesn't mean that you can never have a light beer or a glass of dry wine, but it does mean that alcohol is always a major luxury on any kind of weight-loss diet.

- Keep a close eye on the portion sizes listed on labels. Often what you assume is one serving is really two or three—which means you'll get two or three times as much carbohydrate as you bargained for.

- It's important to know that just because a food says it has "0 grams of carbohydrate" per serving, it doesn't mean that it's carbohydrate free. How can this be? Again, it has to do with portion size. The U.S. federal government standards allow labels to say "0 grams" if the food contains 0.4 grams or less per serving, and "<1 gram" if the food contains 0.9 grams or less per serving. Yet we often use these foods in larger quantities, and the grams add up. A perfect example: A reader of mine wanted to know where the carbs in my Margarita Mix (*500 Low-Carb Recipes*) came from—after all, lime juice, lemon juice, and Splenda all had zero grams of carbohydrate. Only they don't, they all have carbs! They only look like they're carb-free because the serving sizes used on the labels are so small. When in doubt, count 0.5 grams per serving for foods that say 0 grams on the label, and 1 gram for foods that say <1 gram.

- Be aware that there have been more than a few cases of mislabeled "low carb" products that turned out to be a lot higher in carbohydrate than the labels let on. If you add a new product to your diet and you bump up a pound or two, or find yourself hungry and craving, take a closer look—and remember that if it seems too good to be true, it just might be.

- This warning also applies to imported food products. Labeling laws vary from country to country, and much of the world does not include fiber counts in the total carb count on nutrition labels—so if you subtract the fiber count from the total carb count, you'll get an inaccurately low total, and eat more carbohydrate than you meant to.

## Common Sense

- The notion that you can eat unlimited quantities of food so long as you keep the carb count very low has been oversold. It does appear to be true that you can eat more calories on a low-carb diet than you could on a carb-containing diet, and still lose weight, and you certainly never have to go hungry, but that doesn't mean you can eat 10,000 calories a day and still lose weight. Eat when you're hungry, eat enough to feel satisfied, then quit till you're physically hungry again. It's a shame that we even need to be told this, it's so basic, but our society has developed a bad habit of eating for the fun of it, regardless of hunger. Cut it out!

- Americans have been programmed to eat for entertainment—snacking for long periods of time on nutritionally empty junk food, whether they're hungry or not. Low-carb foods are filling, and tend to be calorie-dense, and as a result, there are few low-carb foods that you can nosh on for hours without making yourself ill. If you really must have something to nibble on for hours and hours, your best bet is very low-carb vegetables, like celery and cucumber sticks. Pumpkin and sunflower seeds in the shell are another good choice, because having to open each individual shell slows down your consumption dramatically, and keeps your hands busy, to boot. Better yet, find something else to do for entertainment!

- The heart and soul of your nutritional program, for the rest of your life, should be meat, fish, poultry, eggs and cheese, healthy fats, low-carbohydrate vegetables, low-sugar fruits, and nuts and seeds. You know—food. A sugar-free candy bar or brownie or a bag of low-carb chips is never a substitute for a chicken Caesar salad for lunch. Got it?

# Low-Carbohydrate/
# Sugar-Free Specialty Products

- Roughly half of low-carbohydrate dieters find that diet soda and diet fruit flavored beverages like Crystal Light will slow or stop their weight loss. Many also find that these beverages act as a "trigger"—something that sets off their carb cravings. Why this should be so is controversial; some theorize that the aspartame is to blame, while others feel that citric acid, widely used as a flavoring in these products, interferes with ketosis. Still others claim that just the taste of sweetness can cause an insulin release, whether there's any sugar involved or not. The actual reason is unimportant—just know that if you're struggling, one of the first places to look is your diet soda consumption.

- Do not make low-carb specialty products a major part of your diet. Low-carb breads, pastas, candy, cookies, protein bars, etc. are flooding onto the market, and they do provide a nice variety. However, most of these products are not as nutritious, healthful, or filling as real food. Furthermore, they're all extremely expensive! And almost all of them have more carbohydrates than a hard-boiled egg or a chicken wing. So stop trying to make your low-carb diet look like your old high-carb diet—that's the diet that got you in trouble in the first place, remember?

- When you hit a plateau, lose the treats. The sugar-free chocolate bars, the low-carb baked goods, etc. are the first things to axe if you're not losing weight.

- Regarding those sugar-free chocolate bars, not to mention protein bars, jelly beans, brownies, etc: Just about all of them are sweetened with polyols, sometimes called sugar alcohols. These are carbohydrates, but they're carbohydrates that are slowly and incompletely absorbed, at most. Because of this, most low-carbers and all low-carb specialty food labels subtract out polyols from the total carb count, just like fiber. Polyol sweetened treats are easier on your body than the sugar sweetened kind, but it's optimistic to assume that none of that carbohydrate is absorbed. When low-carb sweets say you can subtract out all of the sugar alcohols from the carb count, take that with a grain of salt.

- Also be aware that polyols/sugar alcohols will cause gas and/or diarrhea if you eat them in any quantity. Be very careful with your portions—I rarely eat more than a half of a 1.5 ounce chocolate bar in a day. Don't eat sugar-free sweets at all before a big job interview, an important presentation, a hot date, or getting on a plane, or you may well be sorry.

## When You're Away From Home

- Make the best choice possible given any particular circumstance. What do I mean? If you're at work, and the vending machine has cookies, crackers, chips, candy, and peanuts, the peanuts are the best choice, even though they're relatively high carb for a nut (because, of course, they're really a legume!). When you're genuinely hungry, and faced with foods which are not ideal for the diet, choose the food that will screw you up the least. Don't be afraid to pick off breading, eat only the cheese and toppings off the pizza, ask for an extra salad in place of the potato, etc.

- Always remember that restaurants are in a service industry. If you're not certain what's in a dish, ask questions about ingredients. Do not hesitate to ask for low-carb substitutions, within reason—steamed vegetables in place of the potato, a bed of lettuce instead of rice, whatever will make your meal low-carb, delicious, and satisfying. If the waiter or the kitchen gives you grief, go spend your money elsewhere. And if they're nice about it—as most restaurants are—be effusive with your praise, and tip well!

- Be polite but firm with people who want you to cheat on your diet. If you're embarrassed about asking for food exactly the way you want it at a restaurant, or about letting your friends know about your food restrictions before a dinner party, let me ask you this: If you had a deadly allergy, one that would cause you to go into anaphylactic shock and die at the mere taste of the wrong food, would you hesitate to bring it up to a waiter or a friend? Of course not, and no one would expect you to. Take care of yourself. More people die of the effects of carbohydrate intolerance—heart disease, stroke, diabetes, cancer—than die of anything else! Your carbohydrate intolerance is just as deadly as the severest allergy. It just takes longer, that's all. I find that it's often easier to say, "I'm afraid I can't have that" than to say, "Oh, no thanks, I'm on a diet." People are far less likely to argue if you make it sound medical—which it is!

- When you're traveling, carry some "friendly" food in your purse or carry-on bag. With transportation being as flukey as it is, and airlines rarely handing out anything more than pretzels, who knows how hungry you could get? Carry individually wrapped string cheese, a protein bar or two, some Just-The-Cheese Chips, a packet or two of nuts or seeds—anything that will get you through if the interval between meals gets stretched out unbearably.

## 10 Great Snacks for 5 grams of Usable Carb—Or Less!

- **Cinnamon and Splenda flavored pork rinds,\* 0.5 ounces:** 2 grams carb, 0 grams fiber, 2 grams usable carb, 6 grams protein, 80 calories.
  *\* Gram's Gourmet makes these.*

- **Cheddar pork rinds,\* 0.5 ounces:** 2 grams carb, 0 grams fiber, 2 grams usable carb, 6 grams protein, 80 calories.
  *\* Gram's Gourmet calls them Cheddar Cheese Crunchies.*

- **Hard-boiled egg:\*** 0.5 grams carb, 0 grams fiber, 0.5 grams usable carb, 6 grams protein, 77 calories.
  *\* Turning that egg into a deviled egg with a little mayo and mustard will add less than 1 gram of carbohydrate!*

- **Frozen hot wings,\* 4 pieces:** 1 gram carb, 0 grams fiber, 1 gram usable carb, 20 grams protein, 220 calories.
  *\* Not barbecue wings—barbecue sauce is sugary.*

- **1/3 cup smoke-flavored roasted almonds:** 8 grams carb, 4 grams fiber, 4 grams usable carb, 12 grams protein, 360 calories.

- **1 ounce blue cheese and 1 ounce cream cheese, mashed together and stuffed into 1 large celery rib:** 3 grams carb, 1 gram fiber, 2 grams usable carb, 9 grams protein, 205 calories.

- **1 ounce pumpkin seeds:\*** 4 grams carb, 2 grams fiber, 2 grams usable carb, 9 grams protein, 150 calories.
  *\* Pumpkorn brand comes in great flavors!*

- **1 ounce deluxe mixed nuts (w/o peanuts):** 6 grams carb, 1 gram fiber, 5 grams usable carb, 4 grams protein, 174 calories.

- **String cheese, 2 snack-sized sticks:** 0 grams carb, 0 grams fiber, 0 grams usable carb, 14 grams protein, 160 calories.

- Hot dog (No bun of course!) The most common brand
  (Oscar Meyer): 1 gram carb, 0 grams fiber, 1 gram usable
  carb, 5.1 grams protein, 147 calories.

## 10 Treats for 10 Grams or Less

- **Sugar-free ice pop, 1 stick:** 3.5 grams carb, 0 grams fiber,
  3.5 grams usable carb, 0.4 grams protein, 17 calories.

- **6 large strawberries with $1/2$ cup whipped cream (no sugar):**
  7 grams carb, 2 grams fiber, 5 grams usable carb,
  2 grams protein, 228 calories.

- **1 serving sugar-free instant pudding made with half heavy
  cream, half water:** 2 grams carb, 0 grams fiber,
  2 grams usable carb, 1 gram protein, 205 calories.

- **$1/8$ medium cantaloupe, sprinkled with 1 tablespoon lime
  juice and $1/2$ tablespoon Splenda:** 8 grams carb,
  1 gram fiber, 7 grams usable carb, 1 gram protein, 31 calories.

- **Sugar-free fudge pop, 1 stick:** 9 grams carb, 0 grams fiber, 9
  grams usable carb, 2 grams protein, 45 calories.

- **2 cups popcorn:** 12 grams carb, 2 grams fiber, 10 grams usable carb, <1 gram protein, 55 calories (assuming oil popped).

- **$1/2$ bag Keto brand low carb Nacho Cheese Tortilla Chips:**
  16 grams carb, 8 grams fiber, 8 grams usable carb, 24 grams
  protein, 300 calories.

- **$3/4$ cup plain yogurt with ½ teaspoon vanilla extract,
  1 tablespoon Splenda, and ¼ cup Gram's Flax 'n' Nut
  Crunchies\* stirred in:** 8 grams carb, 3 grams fiber, 5 grams
  usable carb, 12 grams protein, 301 calories.

* *This is a low carb granola-like product made of nuts and seeds.*

- **5 Reese's miniature sugar-free peanut butter cups:**
  23 grams carb, 1 gram fiber, 19 grams polyols, 3 grams
  usable carb, 2 grams protein, 170 calories.

- **17 Jelly Belly sugar free jelly beans:\*** 18 grams carb,
  0 grams fiber, 16 grams polyols, 2 grams usable carb, 0 grams
  protein, 60 calories.
  *\*This is half of what the Jelly Belly company lists as a serving
  size, but since these are so polyol-rich, I fear that eating 35 jelly
  beans would cause gastric upset in many people. Be warned!*

## Lowest-Carb Fast Food Meals

For a more complete list of fast food that will work for a low-
carb diet, see page 104—these are just the very lowest-carb
choices at each of the biggest chains. Your beverage choices
will be coffee, tea, iced tea, diet soda, or water.

### Arby's
**Asian Sesame Salad:** 15 grams carb, 3 grams fiber,
12 grams usable carb, 18 grams protein, 140 calories.

### Burger King
**Chicken Whopper, Low-carb:** 3 grams carb, 1 gram fiber,
2 grams usable carb, 30 grams protein, 160 calories.

### Boston Market
**Marinated Grilled Chicken:** 1 gram carb, 0 grams fiber,
1 gram usable carb, 33 grams protein, 230 calories.

### Hardee's
**1/3 Pound (pre-cooked weight) Low-carb Thickburger:**
5 grams carb, 2 grams fiber, 3 grams usable carb, 30 grams
protein, 420 calories.

### McDonalds
**Caesar Salad:** 7 grams carb, 3 grams fiber, 4 grams usable
carb, 7 grams protein, 90 calories.

**California Cobb Salad:** 7 grams carb, 3 grams fiber, 4 grams usable carb, 11 grams protein, 150 calories.

**Dressings:** Newman's Own Creamy Caesar, 4 grams carb, 0 grams fiber, 4 grams usable carb, 2 grams protein, 190 calories; or Low-Fat Balsamic Vinaigrette, 4 grams carb, 0 grams fiber, 4 grams usable carb, 0 grams protein, 40 calories.

### Pizza Hut

**Hot Wings, 4 pieces:** 2 grams carb, 0 grams fiber, 2 grams usable carb, 22 grams protein, 220 calories.

**Mild Wings, 4 pieces:** <2 grams carb, 0 grams fiber, <2 grams usable carb, 22 grams protein, 220 calories.

### Steak-N-Shake

**Chicken Chef Salad:** 11 grams carb, 3 grams fiber, 8 grams usable carb, 36 grams protein, 472 calories.

### Subway

Aside from the omelets, which are 2 to 3 grams of usable carb each and roughly 20 grams protein...

**Grilled Chicken and Spinach Salad:** 11 grams carb, 5 grams fiber, 6 grams usable carb, 39 grams protein, 620 calories.

### Taco Bell

**Taco Salad, no beans, no shell, double chicken:** 15 grams carb, 4 grams fiber, 11 grams usable carb, 43 grams protein, 452 calories.

### Wendy's

**Chicken BLT Salad:** 10 grams carb, 4 grams fiber, 6 grams usable carb, 34 grams protein, 310 calories.

# How to Use This Book

This book is designed to help you count calories and nutrients accurately, quickly, and easily. Alphabetical listings make locating your foods simple. To improve clarity and speed in locating food choices, this book is divided into 3 sections:

> **Beverages**
>
> **Foods**
>
> **Fast Food Restaurants**

## Abbreviation Key

| | | | |
|---|---|---|---|
| appx | *approximately* | mg | *milligram(s)* |
| as prep | *prepared as instructed on package, usual method* | ml | *milliliter* |
| | | oz | *ounce* |
| | | pkg | *package* |
| avg | *average size* | pkt | *packet* |
| bev | *beverage* | prep | *prepared* |
| cal | *calorie* | sm | *small* |
| dia | *diameter* | svg | *serving* |
| fl oz | *fluid ounce* | sq | *square* |
| g | *gram(s)* | Tbsp | *tablespoon* |
| " | *inch(es)* | Tr | *trace—less than 1 g or mg* |
| Lb | *pound* | | |
| Lg | *large* | tsp | *teaspoon* |
| mcg | *microgram* | w/ | *with* |
| med | *medium* | w/o | *without* |
| misc | *miscellaneous* | | |

# Please Note

- All listings are medium- or average-portion size, unless specifically noted.

- "Cooked" means the food is cooked without added fats, sauces, or sugars. This includes boiling, steaming, and heating in a microwave oven.

- "Baked" and "broiled" describe the normal methods of baking and broiling, without oil, or minimal cooking oil for a non-stick surface. No other fats, sauces, or sugars added.

- Net carbs are taken from the manufacturers' nutritional information, or calculated by subtracting fiber from total carbs. Net carbs are rounded to whole numbers.

- Food entries with less than 5 grams net carb per serving are in BOLD.

- The data is accurate at the time publication. However, food manufacturers may change their ingredients at any time without notice. Food nutrition labels should also be checked. Keep your eyes open for new low-carb products!

### References for compiling this book:

- The United States Department of Agriculture (USDA) nutritional database (2002)

- Food manufacturers' nutrient labels (2004)

- Restaurants' printed nutritional data (2004)

# BEVERAGES

(See Food and Fast Food Restaurants listed separately)

| | Serving Size | Calories (g) | Total Carbs(g) | Fiber (g) | Net Carbs(g) | Protein (g) | Fat (g) |
|---|---|---|---|---|---|---|---|
| **Amaretto, 53 proof** | 1.5 fl oz | 175 | 24 | 0 | 24 | Tr | Tr |
| **Apple Juice** | 8 fl oz | 115 | 29 | Tr | 29 | Tr | Tr |
| **Apple-Cranberry Juice** | 8 fl oz | 115 | 29 | Tr | 29 | Tr | Tr |
| **Apple-Grape Juice** | 8 fl oz | 130 | 31 | Tr | 31 | Tr | Tr |
| **Apple-Raspberry Juice** | 8 fl oz | 120 | 30 | Tr | 30 | Tr | Tr |
| **Apricot Nectar** | 8 fl oz | 140 | 36 | Tr | 36 | Tr | Tr |
| **Beer** | | | | | | | |
| Regular beer | 12 fl oz | 150 | 13 | 1 | 12 | 1 | 0 |
| Light beer | 12 fl oz | 100 | 6 | 0 | 6 | 1 | 0 |
| Dark beer | 12 fl oz | 160 | 14 | Tr | 14 | 1 | 0 |
| Draft beer, regular | 12 fl oz | 150 | 13 | Tr | 13 | 1 | 0 |
| Draft beer, light | 12 fl oz | 100 | 6 | 0 | 6 | 1 | 0 |
| Dry beer | 12 fl oz | 130 | 8 | Tr | 8 | 1 | 0 |
| Malt beer | 12 fl oz | 160 | 10 | Tr | 10 | 1 | 0 |
| **Bloody Mary** | 5 fl oz | 150 | 5 | Tr | 5 | 1 | Tr |
| **Bourbon** | | | | | | | |
| *80 proof* | *1.5 fl oz* | *95* | *0* | *0* | *0* | *0* | *0* |
| *86 proof* | *1.5 fl oz* | *105* | *Tr* | *0* | *Tr* | *0* | *0* |
| *90 proof* | *1.5 fl oz* | *110* | *Tr* | *0* | *Tr* | *0* | *0* |
| **Brandy** | | | | | | | |
| *80 proof* | *1.5 fl oz* | *95* | *0* | *0* | *0* | *0* | *0* |
| *86 proof* | *1.5 fl oz* | *105* | *Tr* | *0* | *Tr* | *0* | *0* |
| *90 proof* | *1.5 fl oz* | *110* | *Tr* | *0* | *Tr* | *0* | *0* |
| Flavored, 60 proof (Apricot Blackberry, Cherry, or Coffee) | 1.5 fl oz | 180 | 24 | 0 | 24 | Tr | Tr |
| *Capri Sun* juice drink | 8 fl oz | 122 | 31 | Tr | 31 | Tr | Tr |
| **Carbonated Beverages** see Soda | | | | | | | |
| Carrot Juice | 8 fl oz | 95 | 22 | 2 | 20 | 2 | Tr |
| ***Club Soda*** | ***12 fl oz*** | ***0*** | ***0*** | ***0*** | ***0*** | ***0*** | ***0*** |

| | Serving Size | Calories (g) | Total Carbs(g) | Fiber (g) | Net Carbs(g) | Protein (g) | Fat (g) |
|---|---|---|---|---|---|---|---|
| **Cocoa/Chocolate Beverage, Hot** | | | | | | | |
| Regular, as prep | 6 fl oz | 170 | 23 | 1 | 22 | 7 | 7 |
| Diet or sugar-free, as prep | 6 fl oz | 35 | 5 | Tr | 5 | 3 | 0 |
| **Coffee** | | | | | | | |
| ***Brewed coffee, regular or decaf*** | ***6 fl oz*** | ***4*** | ***1*** | ***0*** | ***1*** | ***Tr*** | ***0*** |
| ***Instant coffee, regular or decaf*** | ***6 fl oz*** | ***4*** | ***1*** | ***0*** | ***1*** | ***Tr*** | ***0*** |
| Café Amaretto | 6 fl oz | 70 | 6 | 0 | 6 | 7 | 2 |
| Café Latte | 6 fl oz | 115 | 10 | 0 | 10 | 6 | 6 |
| Café Vienna | 6 fl oz | 70 | 6 | 0 | 6 | 7 | 2 |
| Cappuccino | 6 fl oz | 65 | 6 | 0 | 6 | 3 | 3 |
| ***Espresso*** | ***2 fl oz*** | ***5*** | ***1*** | ***0*** | ***1*** | ***Tr*** | ***Tr*** |
| French Vanilla Café | 6 fl oz | 70 | 6 | 0 | 6 | 7 | 2 |
| ***French Vanilla, sugar-free*** | ***6 fl oz*** | ***20*** | ***4*** | ***0*** | ***4*** | ***Tr*** | ***Tr*** |
| Hazelnut Belgian Café | 6 fl oz | 75 | 7 | 0 | 7 | 7 | 2 |
| Swiss Mocha coffee | 6 fl oz | 75 | 8 | Tr | 8 | 9 | 1 |
| ***Swiss Mocha coffee, sugar-free*** | ***6 fl oz*** | ***20*** | ***4*** | ***0*** | ***4*** | ***Tr*** | ***Tr*** |
| Viennese Chocolate coffee | 6 fl oz | 75 | 8 | Tr | 8 | 9 | 1 |
| **Coffee Cream – see Creamer** | ... | ... | . | . | . | . | . |
| **Coffee Liqueur, 53 proof** | 1.5 fl oz | 175 | 24 | 0 | 24 | Tr | Tr |
| **Coke - see Soda** | ... | ... | . | . | . | . | . |
| **Cola - see Soda** | ... | ... | . | . | . | . | . |
| **Cranapple Drink** | 8 fl oz | 170 | 43 | Tr | 43 | 0 | 0 |
| **Cranberry Juice Cocktail** | 8 fl oz | 145 | 36 | Tr | 36 | 0 | Tr |
| **Cranberry-Grape Drink** | 8 fl oz | 145 | 34 | Tr | 34 | Tr | Tr |
| **Creamer** | | | | | | | |
| ***Half & Half (cream & milk)*** | ***1 Tbsp*** | ***20*** | ***1*** | ***0*** | ***1*** | ***1*** | ***2*** |
| Half & Half (cream & milk) | 1 cup | 315 | 10 | 0 | 10 | 7 | 28 |
| ***Liquid creamer Coffee-Mate*** | ***1 Tbsp*** | ***20*** | ***2*** | ***0*** | ***2*** | ***Tr*** | ***1*** |
| ***Powdered creamer Coffee-Mate*** | ***1 tsp*** | ***10*** | ***2*** | ***0*** | ***2*** | ***Tr*** | ***Tr*** |

| | Serving Size | Calories (g) | Total Carbs(g) | Fiber (g) | Net Carbs(g) | Protein (g) | Fat (g) |
|---|---|---|---|---|---|---|---|
| Crème de Menthe | 1 fl oz | 125 | 14 | 0 | 14 | 0 | 0 |
| *Crystal Light, all flavors* | *8 fl oz* | *5* | *0* | *0* | *0* | *0* | *0* |
| Daiquiri, strawberry | 4 fl oz | 225 | 8 | Tr | 8 | Tr | Tr |
| *Diet Cola* | *12 fl oz* | *0* | *0* | *0* | *0* | *0* | *0* |
| Eggnog, plain | 1 cup | 345 | 34 | 0 | 34 | 10 | 19 |
| Fruit Drink (5% to 10% juice) Cherry, Grape, Orange, or Strawberry | | | | | | | |
| Regular | 8 fl oz | 135 | 32 | Tr | 32 | 0 | 0 |
| *Sugar-free* | *8 fl oz* | *5* | *1* | *Tr* | *1* | *0* | *0* |
| Fruit Punch (10% Juice) | | | | | | | |
| Regular | 8 fl oz | 130 | 31 | Tr | 31 | 0 | 0 |
| *Sugar-free* | *8 fl oz* | *5* | *1* | *Tr* | *1* | *0* | *0* |
| Gatorade | 8 fl oz | 50 | 14 | 0 | 14 | 0 | 0 |
| Gin | | | | | | | |
| *80 proof* | *1.5 fl oz* | *95* | *0* | *0* | *0* | *0* | *0* |
| *86 proof* | *1.5 fl oz* | *105* | *Tr* | *0* | *Tr* | *0* | *0* |
| *90 proof* | *1.5 fl oz* | *110* | *Tr* | *0* | *Tr* | *0* | *0* |
| Grape Juice | | | | | | | |
| Canned or bottled, sweetened | 8 fl oz | 155 | 38 | Tr | 38 | 1 | Tr |
| Frozen concentrate, sweetened as prep w/ water | 8 fl oz | 130 | 32 | Tr | 32 | Tr | Tr |
| Unsweetened grape juice | 8 fl oz | 120 | 30 | Tr | 30 | Tr | Tr |
| Grapefruit Juice | | | | | | | |
| Fresh, squeezed, unsweetened | 8 fl oz | 95 | 22 | Tr | 22 | 1 | Tr |
| Fresh, squeezed, sugar sweetened | 8 fl oz | 115 | 28 | Tr | 28 | 1 | Tr |
| Fresh, squeezed, w/ aspartame | 8 fl oz | 95 | 22 | Tr | 22 | 1 | Tr |
| Canned, unsweetened | 8 fl oz | 95 | 22 | Tr | 22 | 1 | Tr |
| Canned, sugar sweetened | 8 fl oz | 115 | 28 | Tr | 28 | 1 | Tr |
| Frozen concentrate, unsweetened, as prep w/ water | 8 fl oz | 100 | 24 | Tr | 24 | 1 | Tr |

| | Serving Size | Calories (g) | Total Carbs(g) | Fiber (g) | Net Carbs(g) | Protein (g) | Fat (g) |
|---|---|---|---|---|---|---|---|
| *Half & Half* – see Creamer | ... | ... | . | . | . | . | . |
| *Hawaiian Punch* | | | | | | | |
| Regular | 8 fl oz | 120 | 30 | Tr | 30 | 0 | 0 |
| *Sugar-free* | *8 fl oz* | *15* | *4* | *Tr* | *4* | *0* | *0* |
| Hot Cocoa/Chocolate – see Cocoa | ... | ... | . | . | . | . | . |
| Juice – see specific listings | ... | ... | . | . | . | . | . |
| *Kool Aid* | | | | | | | |
| Sugar sweetened | 8 fl oz | 60 | 16 | Tr | 16 | 0 | 0 |
| *Sugar-free* | *8 fl oz* | *5* | *1* | *Tr* | *1* | *0* | *0* |
| *Unsweetened Packet* | *1 pkt* | *0* | *0* | *0* | *0* | *0* | *0* |
| Lemon Juice | | | | | | | |
| *Fresh, squeezed, unsweetened* | *1 Tbsp* | *4* | *1* | *Tr* | *1* | *Tr* | *Tr* |
| *Canned or bottled, unsweetened* | *1 Tbsp* | *3* | *1* | *Tr* | *1* | *Tr* | *Tr* |
| Canned or bottled, unsweetened | 1 cup | 50 | 16 | 1 | 15 | 1 | 1 |
| Lemonade | | | | | | | |
| Sugar Sweetened | 8 fl oz | 100 | 25 | Tr | 25 | 0 | 0 |
| *Sugar-free* | *8 fl oz* | *5* | *1* | *Tr* | *1* | *0* | *0* |
| Lime Juice | | | | | | | |
| *Fresh or bottled, unsweetened* | *1 Tbsp* | *3* | *1* | *Tr* | *1* | *Tr* | *Tr* |
| Fresh or bottled, unsweetened | 1 cup | 52 | 16 | 1 | 15 | 1 | 1 |
| Limeade | | | | | | | |
| Sugar sweetened | 8 fl oz | 100 | 25 | Tr | 25 | 0 | 0 |
| *Sugar-free* | *8 fl oz* | *5* | *1* | *Tr* | *1* | *0* | *0* |
| Liqueur, 53 proof | | | | | | | |
| Coffee or Fruit Flavored | 1.5 fl oz | 175 | 24 | 0 | 24 | Tr | Tr |
| Mai Tai | 5 fl oz | 280 | 28 | 1 | 27 | 1 | Tr |
| Margarita | 5 fl oz | 150 | 10 | Tr | 10 | 0 | 0 |
| *Martini* | *2.5 fl oz* | *155* | *0* | *0* | *0* | *0* | *0* |
| Milk | | | | | | | |
| **White Milk** | | | | | | | |
| Whole milk, 3.3% fat | 8 fl oz | 150 | 11 | 0 | 11 | 8 | 8 |

| | Serving Size | Calories (g) | Total Carbs(g) | Fiber (g) | Net Carbs(g) | Protein (g) | Fat (g) |
|---|---|---|---|---|---|---|---|
| Reduced fat milk, 2%fat | 8 fl oz | 120 | 12 | 0 | 12 | 8 | 5 |
| Lowfat milk, 1% fat | 8 fl oz | 102 | 12 | 0 | 12 | 8 | 3 |
| Nonfat milk, (Skim milk) | 8 fl oz | 85 | 12 | 0 | 12 | 8 | Tr |
| Nonfat instant, as prep w/water | 8 fl oz | 80 | 12 | 0 | 12 | 8 | 0 |
| Nonfat instant, dry powder only | 1 cup | 240 | 36 | 0 | 36 | 24 | 0 |
| **Chocolate Milk** | | | | | | | |
| Whole chocolate milk | 8 fl oz | 210 | 26 | 2 | 24 | 8 | 8 |
| Reduced fat chocolate milk, 2% | 8 fl oz | 180 | 26 | 1 | 25 | 8 | 5 |
| Lowfat chocolate milk, 1% | 8 fl oz | 160 | 26 | 1 | 25 | 8 | 3 |
| **Misc Milk Products** | | | | | | | |
| Buttermilk | 1 cup | 100 | 12 | 0 | 12 | 8 | 2 |
| Condensed, sweetened | 1 cup | 980 | 166 | 0 | 166 | 24 | 27 |
| Evaporated whole milk | 1 cup | 340 | 25 | 0 | 25 | 17 | 19 |
| Evaporated skim milk | 1 cup | 200 | 29 | 0 | 29 | 19 | 1 |
| Malted milk, chocolate | 1 cup | 225 | 29 | Tr | 29 | 9 | 9 |
| Malted milk, natural | 1 cup | 230 | 28 | 0 | 28 | 10 | 9 |
| *Soy milk* | *1 cup* | *81* | *4* | *3* | *1* | *7* | *5* |
| **Milk Shake** – see Shake | ... | ... | . | . | . | . | . |
| **Miso** | 1 cup | 567 | 77 | 15 | 62 | 32 | 17 |
| *Nesquik*, Chocolate, as prep | 8 fl oz | 210 | 33 | 1 | 32 | 7 | 5 |
| **Orange Juice** | | | | | | | |
| Fresh, squeezed, unsweetened | 8 fl oz | 112 | 26 | 1 | 25 | 2 | Tr |
| Canned or bottled, unsweetened | 8 fl oz | 110 | 25 | 1 | 24 | 2 | Tr |
| Frozen concentrate, as prep | 8 fl oz | 112 | 26 | 1 | 25 | 2 | Tr |
| **Peach Nectar** | 8 fl oz | 135 | 34 | Tr | 34 | 1 | 0 |
| **Pear Nectar** | 8 fl oz | 150 | 39 | Tr | 39 | 0 | 0 |
| **Pepsi** – see Soda | ... | ... | . | . | . | . | . |
| **Pina Colada** | 4.5 fl oz | 260 | 40 | 1 | 39 | 1 | 3 |
| **Pineapple Grapefruit Juice** | 8 fl oz | 120 | 29 | Tr | 29 | 1 | Tr |

| | Serving Size | Calories (g) | Total Carbs(g) | Fiber (g) | Net Carbs(g) | Protein (g) | Fat (g) |
|---|---|---|---|---|---|---|---|
| Pineapple Juice | 8 fl oz | 140 | 34 | 1 | 33 | 1 | Tr |
| Pineapple Orange Juice | 8 fl oz | 125 | 30 | Tr | 30 | 3 | 0 |
| Prune Juice | 8 fl oz | 182 | 45 | 3 | 42 | 2 | Tr |
| **Root Beer** | | | | | | | |
| Regular | 12 fl oz | 170 | 47 | 0 | 47 | 0 | 0 |
| *Diet or sugar-free* | *12 fl oz* | *0* | *0* | *0* | *0* | *0* | *0* |
| **Rum** | | | | | | | |
| *80 proof* | *1.5 fl oz* | *95* | *0* | *0* | *0* | *0* | *0* |
| *86 proof* | *1.5 fl oz* | *105* | *Tr* | *0* | *Tr* | *0* | *0* |
| *90 proof* | *1.5 fl oz* | *110* | *Tr* | *0* | *Tr* | *0* | *0* |
| **Scotch** | | | | | | | |
| *80 proof* | *1.5 fl oz* | *95* | *0* | *0* | *0* | *0* | *0* |
| *86 proof* | *1.5 fl oz* | *105* | *Tr* | *0* | *Tr* | *0* | *0* |
| *90 proof* | *1.5 fl oz* | *110* | *Tr* | *0* | *Tr* | *0* | *0* |
| Screwdriver | 7 fl oz | 160 | 17 | 1 | 16 | Tr | Tr |
| **Shake** | | | | | | | |
| Regular milk shake | | | | | | | |
| Chocolate | 11 oz | 360 | 63 | 1 | 62 | 9 | 8 |
| Peach | 11 oz | 380 | 75 | 1 | 74 | 10 | 4 |
| Strawberry | 11 oz | 395 | 80 | 1 | 79 | 11 | 4 |
| Vanilla | 11 Oz | 350 | 56 | 0 | 56 | 12 | 9 |
| Low carb shake | | | | | | | |
| *Atkins chocolate shake* | *11 oz* | *170* | *5* | *3* | *2* | *20* | *9* |
| *Atkins vanilla shake* | *11 oz* | *170* | *4* | *2* | *2* | *20* | *9* |
| **Soda / Cola / Soft Drink** *(Carbonated Beverages)* | | | | | | | |
| *Club Soda* | *12 fl oz* | *0* | *0* | *0* | *0* | *0* | *0* |
| Cherry Cola, regular | 12 fl oz | 155 | 40 | 0 | 40 | 0 | 0 |
| *Cherry Cola, diet* | *12 fl oz* | *0* | *0* | *0* | *0* | *0* | *0* |
| Coca Cola, Coke regular | 12 fl oz | 140 | 39 | 0 | 39 | 0 | 0 |
| *Coke, diet* | *12 fl oz* | *0* | *0* | *0* | *0* | *0* | *0* |
| Cola | 12 fl oz | 150 | 40 | 0 | 40 | 0 | 0 |
| *Diet Cola* | *12 fl oz* | *0* | *0* | *0* | *0* | *0* | *0* |
| *Dr Pepper, regular* | 12 fl oz | 150 | 40 | 0 | 40 | 0 | 0 |
| *Dr Pepper, diet* | *12 fl oz* | *0* | *0* | *0* | *0* | *0* | *0* |
| Ginger Ale, regular | 12 fl oz | 125 | 32 | 0 | 32 | 0 | 0 |
| *Ginger Ale, diet* | *12 fl oz* | *0* | *0* | *0* | *0* | *0* | *0* |
| Grape Soda, regular | 12 fl oz | 155 | 40 | 0 | 40 | 0 | 0 |

| | Serving Size | Calories (g) | Total Carbs(g) | Fiber (g) | Net Carbs(g) | Protein (g) | Fat (g) |
|---|---|---|---|---|---|---|---|
| *Grape Soda, diet* | *12 fl oz* | *0* | *0* | *0* | *0* | *0* | *0* |
| Lemon Lime Soda, regular | 12 fl oz | 145 | 36 | 0 | 36 | 0 | 0 |
| *Lemon Lime Soda, diet* | *12 fl oz* | *0* | *0* | *0* | *0* | *0* | *0* |
| *Mountain Dew, regular* | 12 fl oz | 170 | 46 | 0 | 46 | 0 | 0 |
| *Mountain Dew, diet* | *12 fl oz* | *0* | *0* | *0* | *0* | *0* | *0* |
| *Mr. Pibb, regular* | 12 fl oz | 146 | 39 | 0 | 39 | 0 | 0 |
| *Mr. Pibb, diet* | *12 fl oz* | *0* | *0* | *0* | *0* | *0* | *0* |
| Orange Soda, regular | 12 fl oz | 175 | 45 | 0 | 45 | 0 | 0 |
| *Orange Soda, diet* | *12 fl oz* | *0* | *0* | *0* | *0* | *0* | *0* |
| *Pepsi, regular* | 12 fl oz | 150 | 41 | 0 | 41 | 0 | 0 |
| *Pepsi, diet* | *12 fl oz* | *0* | *0* | *0* | *0* | *0* | *0* |
| *RC Cola, regular* | 12 fl oz | 160 | 43 | 0 | 43 | 0 | 0 |
| *RC Cola, diet* | *12 fl oz* | *0* | *0* | *0* | *0* | *0* | *0* |
| Root Beer, Regular | 12 fl oz | 170 | 44 | 0 | 44 | 0 | 0 |
| *Root Beer, Diet* | *12 fl oz* | *0* | *0* | *0* | *0* | *0* | *0* |
| *Seven Up, regular* | 12 fl oz | 150 | 39 | 0 | 39 | 0 | 0 |
| *Seven Up, diet* | *12 fl oz* | *0* | *0* | *0* | *0* | *0* | *0* |
| *Sprite, regular* | 12 fl oz | 150 | 39 | 0 | 39 | 0 | 0 |
| *Sprite, diet* | *12 fl oz* | *0* | *0* | *0* | *0* | *0* | *0* |
| *Tab* | *12 fl oz* | *1* | *0* | *0* | *0* | *0* | *0* |
| Soft Drinks – see Soda | ... | ... | . | . | . | . | . |
| Sport Drink | 12 fl oz | 75 | 18 | 0 | 18 | 0 | 0 |
| Sugar-free Beverage (Also see specific listings) | | | | | | | |
| *Sugar-free Soda* | *12 fl oz* | *0* | *0* | *0* | *0* | *0* | *0* |
| *Sugar-free Kool Aid* | *8 fl oz* | *5* | *1* | *Tr* | *1* | *0* | *0* |
| Sunny Delight, Citrus Punch | 8 fl oz | 125 | 31 | Tr | 31 | 0 | 0 |
| Tang, regular | 8 fl oz | 115 | 29 | Tr | 29 | 0 | 0 |
| *Tang, sugar-free* | *8 fl oz* | *5* | *Tr* | *Tr* | *Tr* | *0* | *0* |
| Tea, Hot or Iced | | | | | | | |
| *Regular, unsweetened* | *8 fl oz* | *2* | *1* | *0* | *1* | *0* | *0* |
| Regular, sugar sweetened | 8 fl oz | 90 | 22 | 0 | 22 | 0 | 0 |
| *Regular, aspartame sweetened* | *8 fl oz* | *4* | *1* | *0* | *1* | *0* | *0* |
| *Chamomile tea, unsweetened* | *8 fl oz* | *2* | *Tr* | *0* | *Tr* | *0* | *0* |
| Chamomile tea, sugar sweetened | 8 fl oz | 90 | 21 | 0 | 21 | 0 | 0 |

| | Serving Size | Calories (g) | Total Carbs(g) | Fiber (g) | Net Carbs(g) | Protein (g) | Fat (g) |
|---|---|---|---|---|---|---|---|
| Misc Types of Tea, Blends, Black, Chinese, Orange Pekoe | | | | | | | |
| **Unsweetened** | **8 fl oz** | **2** | **Tr** | **0** | **Tr** | **0** | **0** |
| Sugar sweetened | 8 fl oz | 90 | 22 | 0 | 22 | 0 | 0 |
| **Sweetened w/aspartame** | **8 fl oz** | **4** | **1** | **0** | **1** | **0** | **0** |
| **Tequila** | **1.5 fl oz** | **100** | **0** | **0** | **0** | **0** | **0** |
| Tequila Sunrise | 5.5 fl oz | 190 | 15 | 1 | 14 | 1 | 0 |
| Tomato Juice | 8 fl oz | 41 | 10 | 1 | 9 | 2 | Tr |
| V 8 Vegetable Juice, 1 Lg can | 11.5 fl oz | 70 | 15 | 2 | 13 | 2 | 0 |
| Vegetable Juice | 8 fl oz | 46 | 11 | 2 | 9 | 2 | Tr |
| Vodka | | | | | | | |
| **80 proof** | **1.5 fl oz** | **95** | **0** | **0** | **0** | **0** | **0** |
| **86 proof** | **1.5 fl oz** | **105** | **Tr** | **0** | **Tr** | **0** | **0** |
| **90 proof** | **1.5 fl oz** | **110** | **Tr** | **0** | **Tr** | **0** | **0** |
| **Water** | **8 fl oz** | **0** | **0** | **0** | **0** | **0** | **0** |
| Whiskey | | | | | | | |
| **80 proof** | **1.5 fl oz** | **95** | **0** | **0** | **0** | **0** | **0** |
| **86 proof** | **1.5 fl oz** | **105** | **Tr** | **0** | **Tr** | **0** | **0** |
| **90 proof** | **1.5 fl oz** | **110** | **Tr** | **0** | **Tr** | **0** | **0** |
| Wine | | | | | | | |
| Dessert Wine, Dry | 4 fl oz | 150 | 5 | 0 | 5 | Tr | 0 |
| Dessert Wine, Sweet | 4 fl oz | 180 | 14 | 0 | 14 | Tr | 0 |
| **Red Wine (table wine)** | **4 fl oz** | **85** | **2** | **0** | **2** | **Tr** | **0** |
| **Rosè Wine** | **4 fl oz** | **85** | **1** | **0** | **1** | **Tr** | **0** |
| **White Wine (table wine)** | **4 fl oz** | **80** | **1** | **0** | **1** | **Tr** | **0** |
| **White Zinfandel** | **4 fl oz** | **85** | **1** | **0** | **1** | **Tr** | **0** |
| Wine Cooler | 5.5 fl oz | 100 | 11 | 0 | 11 | Tr | 0 |
| **Wine Spritzer** | **5.5 fl oz** | **60** | **1** | **0** | **1** | **Tr** | **0** |

## FOOD
(See Beverages and Fast Food Restaurants listed separately)

| | Serving Size | Calories (g) | Total Carbs(g) | Fiber (g) | Net Carbs(g) | Protein (g) | Fat (g) |
|---|---|---|---|---|---|---|---|
| **Accent Seasoning** | **¼ tsp** | **Tr** | **0** | **0** | **0** | **0** | **0** |
| **Alfalfa sprouts, fresh** | **1 cup** | **10** | **1** | **Tr** | **Tr** | **1** | **Tr** |
| Almonds – see Nuts | ... | ... | . | . | | . | . |
| Anchovy – see Fish | ... | ... | . | . | | . | . |
| **Anise Seed** | **1 Tbsp** | **28** | **3** | **1** | **2** | **1** | **1** |
| Apple | | | | | | | |
| Fresh, unpeeled, avg 2 ¾" dia | 1 | 80 | 21 | 4 | 17 | Tr | Tr |
| Fresh, peeled, sliced | 1 cup | 65 | 16 | 2 | 14 | Tr | Tr |
| Dried | 5 rings | 80 | 21 | 3 | 18 | Tr | Tr |
| **Apple Butter** | 1 Tbsp | 30 | 7 | Tr | 7 | Tr | 0 |
| **Apple Pie Filling** | 2 oz can | 85 | 17 | 1 | 16 | 1 | 11 |
| | 1 Tbsp | 40 | 8 | 1 | 7 | Tr | 1 |
| Applesauce | | | | | | | |
| Sweetened | ½ cup | 97 | 25 | 2 | 23 | Tr | Tr |
| Unsweetened | ½ cup | 52 | 14 | 2 | 12 | Tr | Tr |
| Apricot | | | | | | | |
| **Fresh, 1.3 oz** | **1** | **17** | **4** | **1** | **3** | **Tr** | **Tr** |
| Canned, in heavy syrup | 1 cup | 215 | 55 | 4 | 51 | 1 | Tr |
| Canned, in juice | 1 cup | 115 | 30 | 4 | 26 | 2 | Tr |
| Dried, halves | 10 halves | 85 | 22 | 3 | 19 | 1 | Tr |
| **Artichoke**, Globe or French | | | | | | | |
| Fresh, cooked med | 1 | 60 | 13 | 7 | 6 | 4 | Tr |
| Fresh, cooked, drained | 1 cup | 84 | 19 | 9 | 10 | 6 | Tr |
| Jerusalem artichoke, raw, sliced | 1 cup | 114 | 26 | 2 | 24 | 3 | Tr |
| **Arugula, raw** | **½ cup** | **3** | **Tr** | **Tr** | **Tr** | **Tr** | **0** |
| **Asparagus**, cooked | | | | | | | |
| **Fresh spears med** | **4 spears** | **14** | **3** | **1** | **2** | **2** | **Tr** |
| Fresh, chopped pieces | 1 cup | 43 | 8 | 3 | 5 | 5 | 1 |
| **Frozen, spears** | **4 spears** | **17** | **3** | **1** | **2** | **2** | **Tr** |
| Frozen, chopped pieces | 1 cup | 50 | 9 | 3 | 6 | 5 | 1 |

| | Serving Size | Calories (g) | Total Carbs (g) | Fiber (g) | Net Carbs (g) | Protein (g) | Fat (g) |
|---|---|---|---|---|---|---|---|
| **Canned, 5" spears** | **4 spears** | **14** | **2** | **1** | **1** | **2** | **Tr** |
| **Canned, chopped pieces** | **1 cup** | **46** | **6** | **4** | **2** | **5** | **2** |
| **Aspartame Sweetener** | **1 pkt** | **0** | **Tr** | **0** | **Tr** | **0** | **0** |
| Avocado | | | | | | | |
| **California, 1/5 of whole** | **1 oz** | **50** | **2** | **1** | **1** | **1** | **5** |
| **Florida, 1/10 of whole** | **1 oz** | **30** | **3** | **1** | **2** | **Tr** | **3** |
| Bacon – see Pork | ... | ... | . | . | . | . | . |
| **Bacon Bits** | **1 Tbsp** | **31** | **2** | **1** | **1** | **2** | **2** |
| Bagel,  3 ½" dia | | | | | | | |
| Plain | 1 | 150 | 34 | 2 | 32 | 4 | 1 |
| Cinnamon raisin | 1 | 170 | 36 | 2 | 34 | 5 | 1 |
| Egg | 1 | 160 | 34 | 2 | 32 | 5 | 1 |
| Multigrain | 1 | 150 | 33 | 3 | 30 | 5 | 1 |
| **Baking Powder** | **1 tsp** | **2** | **1** | **Tr** | **Tr** | **0** | **0** |
| **Baking Soda** | **1 tsp** | **0** | **0** | **0** | **0** | **0** | **0** |
| **Bamboo Shoots, cooked** | **1 cup** | **25** | **4** | **2** | **2** | **2** | **1** |
| Banana | | | | | | | |
| Fresh, 7" long | 1 | 110 | 28 | 3 | 25 | 1 | 1 |
| Fresh, sliced | 1 cup | 140 | 35 | 4 | 31 | 2 | 1 |
| Banana Split | 1 | 510 | 96 | 4 | 92 | 8 | 12 |
| Barley | | | | | | | |
| Pearled, cooked | 1 cup | 195 | 44 | 6 | 38 | 4 | 1 |
| Pearled, uncooked | 1 cup | 705 | 155 | 31 | 124 | 20 | 2 |
| **Basil, dried spice** | **½ tsp** | **3** | **Tr** | **Tr** | **Tr** | **Tr** | **0** |
| **Bean Sprouts (mung), cooked** | **1 cup** | **30** | **5** | **2** | **3** | **3** | **Tr** |
| BEANS | | | | | | | |
| Plain Beans, cooked w/o fats | | | | | | | |
| Black beans | ½ cup | 115 | 21 | 8 | 13 | 7 | 1 |
| Great Northern beans | ½ cup | 105 | 19 | 6 | 13 | 7 | 1 |
| *Green beans* | *½ cup* | *22* | *5* | *3* | *2* | *1* | *Tr* |
| Kidney, Red beans | ½ cup | 112 | 20 | 7 | 13 | 7 | 1 |
| Lima, large beans | ½ cup | 100 | 17 | 8 | 9 | 7 | 1 |
| Lima, baby lima beans | ½ cup | 95 | 17 | 10 | 7 | 6 | 1 |

| | Serving Size | Calories (g) | Total Carbs(g) | Fiber (g) | Net Carbs(g) | Protein (g) | Fat (g) |
|---|---|---|---|---|---|---|---|
| Pinto beans | ½ cup | 117 | 22 | 7 | 15 | 7 | 1 |
| Soybeans | ½ cup | 135 | 10 | 5 | 5 | 12 | 6 |
| *Wax beans* | *½ cup* | *25* | *5* | *3* | *2* | *1* | *Tr* |
| White beans | ½ cup | 150 | 28 | 6 | 22 | 9 | 1 |
| *Yellow beans* | *½ cup* | *22* | *5* | *3* | *2* | *1* | *Tr* |
| **Misc Bean Dishes,** as prep | | | | | | | |
| Baked beans, plain or vegetarian | ½ cup | 118 | 26 | 6 | 20 | 6 | 1 |
| Baked beans, BBQ style | ½ cup | 180 | 32 | 7 | 25 | 5 | 3 |
| Baked beans w/frankfurters | ½ cup | 185 | 20 | 9 | 11 | 9 | 8 |
| Baked beans w/tomato sauce | ½ cup | 125 | 25 | 6 | 19 | 7 | 2 |
| Baked beans w/sweet sauce | ½ cup | 140 | 27 | 7 | 20 | 7 | 2 |
| Beans w/ pork | ½ cup | 130 | 24 | 6 | 19 | 5 | 2 |
| Black beans w/ rice | ½ cup | 150 | 23 | 5 | 18 | 4 | 5 |
| Green bean casserole | ½ cup | 140 | 13 | 5 | 8 | 3 | 2 |
| *Green beans w/almonds* | *½ cup* | *60* | *8* | *4* | *4* | *3* | *2* |
| Red beans & rice | ½ cup | 130 | 23 | 6 | 17 | 4 | 2 |
| Refried beans | ½ cup | 118 | 20 | 7 | 13 | 7 | 2 |
| **BEEF** Weights for meat w/o bones (Meats as prep: braised, broiled, grilled, simmered, or roasted) | | | | | | | |
| ***Bottom Round,*** *lean & fat* | *3 oz* | *235* | *0* | *0* | *0* | *24* | *14* |
| *lean only* | *3 oz* | *180* | *0* | *0* | *0* | *27* | *7* |
| *Brisket* | *3 oz* | *250* | *0* | *0* | *0* | *23* | *17* |
| *Chuck Blade, lean & fat* | *3 oz* | *295* | *0* | *0* | *0* | *23* | *22* |
| *lean only* | *3 oz* | *215* | *0* | *0* | *0* | *26* | *11* |
| *Corned Beef, canned* | *3 oz* | *215* | *0* | *0* | *0* | *23* | *13* |
| *Dried Beef, chipped* | *1 oz* | *45* | *Tr* | *0* | *Tr* | *8* | *1* |
| *Eye of Round, lean & fat* | *3 oz* | *195* | *0* | *0* | *0* | *23* | *11* |
| *lean only* | *3 oz* | *145* | *0* | *0* | *0* | *25* | *4* |
| *Flank Steak* | *3 oz* | *225* | *0* | *0* | *0* | *23* | *14* |

|  | Serving Size | Calories (g) | Total Carbs(g) | Fiber (g) | Net Carbs(g) | Protein (g) | Fat (g) |
|---|---|---|---|---|---|---|---|
| ***Ground Beef /*** | | | | | | | |
| ***Hamburger meat,*** | | | | | | | |
|    ***regular*** | *3 oz* | *250* | *0* | *0* | *0* | *20* | *18* |
|    ***lean, 79%*** | *3 oz* | *230* | *0* | *0* | *0* | *21* | *16* |
|    ***extra lean, 83%*** | *3 oz* | *220* | *0* | *0* | *0* | *22* | *14* |
| Liver of beef, fried | 3 oz | 185 | 7 | 0 | 7 | 23 | 7 |
| ***Pastrami*** | *2 oz* | *90* | *2* | *Tr* | *2* | *12* | *4* |
| ***Porterhouse Steak*** | *3.5 oz* | *325* | *0* | *0* | *0* | *22* | *26* |
| ***Pot Roast, Chuck*** | *3.5 oz* | *345* | *0* | *0* | *0* | *27* | *26* |
| ***Prime Ribs*** | *3.5 oz* | *400* | *0* | *0* | *0* | *23* | *34* |
| ***Rib Roast, lean & fat*** | *3 oz* | *305* | *0* | *0* | *0* | *19* | *25* |
|    ***lean only*** | *3 oz* | *195* | *0* | *0* | *0* | *23* | *11* |
| ***Roast Beef*** | *3.5 oz* | *290* | *0* | *0* | *0* | *25* | *20* |
| ***Short Ribs*** | *3.5 oz* | *470* | *0* | *0* | *0* | *22* | *42* |
| ***Sirloin Steak,*** | | | | | | | |
|    ***lean & fat*** | *3 oz* | *220* | *0* | *0* | *0* | *24* | *13* |
|    ***lean only*** | *3 oz* | *165* | *0* | *0* | *0* | *26* | *6* |
| ***T-bone Steak,*** | | | | | | | |
|    ***lean & fat*** | *3.5 oz* | *310* | *0* | *0* | *0* | *23* | *23* |
|    ***lean only*** | *3.5 oz* | *250* | *0* | *0* | *0* | *25* | *16* |
| ***Tenderloin Steak/*** | | | | | | | |
|    ***Top Loin*** | *3.5 oz* | *305* | *0* | *0* | *0* | *25* | *22* |
| ***Top Round*** | *3.5 oz* | *215* | *0* | *0* | *0* | *32* | *9* |
|    (Other Beef Products, see: Bologna, Hot Dog, Salami, Sausage & specific entrées) | ... | ... | . | . | . | . | . |
| **Beef & Macaroni** *Healthy Choice, frozen* | 1 pkg | 210 | 33 | 5 | 28 | 14 | 2 |
| **Beef Burgundy,** *Le Menu entrée* | 1 meal | 315 | 12 | 1 | 11 | 25 | 19 |
| ***Beef Jerky, ¾ oz*** | *1* | *80* | *2* | *Tr* | *2* | *7* | *5* |
| **Beef Meals** – see Hamburger Helper for ground beef meals | ... | ... | . | . | . | . | . |
| **Beef Oriental,** *Lean Cuisine* | 1 meal | 270 | 30 | 3 | 27 | 20 | 8 |
| **Beef Patties,** *Banquet entrée* | 1 meal | 180 | 7 | Tr | 7 | 8 | 14 |

| | Serving Size | Calories (g) | Total Carbs(g) | Fiber (g) | Net Carbs(g) | Protein (g) | Fat (g) |
|---|---|---|---|---|---|---|---|
| **Beef Peppercorn,** *Lean Cuisine* | 1 meal | 260 | 32 | 1 | 31 | 16 | 7 |
| **Beef Portabello,** *Lean Cuisine* | 1 meal | 220 | 24 | 1 | 23 | 14 | 7 |
| **Beef Romanoff** | 1 cup | 290 | 28 | 2 | 26 | 20 | 11 |
| **Beef Stew w/ Vegetables** | 1 cup | 215 | 16 | 4 | 12 | 11 | 12 |
| **Beef Stroganoff,** *Stouffers entrée* | 1 meal | 390 | 30 | 1 | 29 | 23 | 20 |
| **Beef Teriyaki** w/vegetables | 1 cup | 250 | 22 | 3 | 19 | 18 | 10 |
| **Beef Tips,** *Healthy Choice entrée* | 1 meal | 260 | 32 | 1 | 31 | 20 | 6 |
| **Beef w/ Broccoli,** Hunan style | 1 cup | 250 | 30 | 3 | 27 | 18 | 8 |
| **Beef w/Vegetables,** Szechuan | 1 cup | 270 | 30 | 3 | 27 | 20 | 8 |
| **Beet Greens,** *chopped, cooked* | *½ cup* | *20* | *4* | *2* | *2* | *2* | *Tr* |
| **Beets** Fresh, cooked, slices | ½ cup | 38 | 8 | 2 | 6 | 2 | Tr |
| *Fresh, cooked, whole beet, 2" dia* | *1 whole* | *22* | *5* | *1* | *4* | *1* | *Tr* |
| Canned, drained, slices | ½ cup | 27 | 6 | 1 | 5 | 1 | Tr |
| *Canned, drained, whole beet* | *1 whole* | *12* | *2* | *Tr* | *2* | *1* | *Tr* |
| **Biscuit,** plain or buttermilk Prep from recipe, 2 ½" dia | 1 | 210 | 27 | 1 | 26 | 4 | 10 |
| Prep from recipe, 4" dia | 1 | 360 | 45 | 2 | 43 | 7 | 16 |
| Refrigerated dough, baked regular 2 ½" dia | 1 | 95 | 13 | Tr | 13 | 2 | 4 |
| reduced fat, 2 ¼" dia | 1 | 65 | 12 | Tr | 12 | 2 | 1 |
| **Blackberries** Fresh | 1 cup | 75 | 18 | 8 | 10 | 1 | 1 |
| Frozen, no sugar added, thawed | 1 cup | 80 | 19 | 8 | 11 | 1 | 1 |
| **Blueberries** Fresh | 1 cup | 80 | 20 | 4 | 16 | 1 | 1 |

| | Serving Size | Calories (g) | Total Carbs(g) | Fiber (g) | Net Carbs(g) | Protein (g) | Fat (g) |
|---|---|---|---|---|---|---|---|
| Frozen, sugar sweetened, thawed | 1 cup | 185 | 50 | 5 | 45 | 1 | Tr |
| **Bologna (thin ⅛" slices)** | | | | | | | |
| **Beef or Pork, regular** | **2 slices** | **180** | **2** | **0** | **2** | **7** | **16** |
| **Beef or Pork, lowfat** | **2 slices** | **110** | **2** | **0** | **2** | **6** | **9** |
| **Beef or Pork, fat free** | **2 slices** | **60** | **3** | **0** | **3** | **8** | **1** |
| **Chicken or Turkey, regular** | **2 slices** | **160** | **2** | **0** | **2** | **7** | **14** |
| **Chicken or Turkey, lowfat** | **2 slices** | **100** | **2** | **0** | **2** | **6** | **8** |
| **Chicken or Turkey, fat free** | **2 slices** | **60** | **3** | **0** | **3** | **8** | **1** |
| Bouillon – see Soup | ... | ... | . | . | . | . | . |
| **Bratwurst, Boars Head** | **1 wurst** | **300** | **0** | **0** | **0** | **19** | **25** |
| **Braunschweiger, 2 avg slices** | **2 oz** | **205** | **2** | **Tr** | **2** | **8** | **18** |
| BREAD (avg ½" thick slice unless noted) | | | | | | | |
| Banana bread, 1 ¼" slice | 1 slice | 195 | 33 | 1 | 32 | 3 | 6 |
| Boston brown | 1 slice | 88 | 20 | 2 | 18 | 2 | 1 |
| *Bran'ola* | 1 slice | 90 | 18 | 2 | 16 | 3 | 2 |
| Bun, frankfurter, 1.4 oz, 5" long | 1 bun | 100 | 18 | 2 | 16 | 3 | 2 |
| Bun, hamburger, 1.4 oz, 3 ½" dia | 1 bun | 100 | 18 | 2 | 16 | 3 | 2 |
| Bun, Lg, 7" long or 4" dia round | 1 bun | 200 | 36 | 4 | 32 | 6 | 4 |
| *Carb Style, Pepperidge Farms* | 1 slice | 60 | 8 | 3 | 5 | 5 | 2 |
| Carrot bread | 1 slice | 200 | 28 | 2 | 26 | 3 | 9 |
| Cinnamon raisin bread | 1 slice | 90 | 18 | 2 | 16 | 2 | 2 |
| Cornbread, 3" x 2" | 1 piece | 185 | 29 | 1 | 28 | 4 | 6 |
| Cracked wheat bread | 1 slice | 65 | 12 | 1 | 11 | 2 | 1 |
| Croissant, butter flavor, 4" | 1 | 230 | 26 | 2 | 24 | 5 | 12 |
| Egg bread, ¾" slice | 1 slice | 115 | 19 | 1 | 18 | 4 | 2 |
| English muffin, regular | 1 whole | 135 | 26 | 2 | 24 | 4 | 1 |
| English muffin, cinnamon/raisin | 1 whole | 140 | 28 | 2 | 26 | 4 | 2 |
| French bread | 1 slice | 70 | 13 | 1 | 12 | 2 | 1 |

| | Serving Size | Calories (g) | Total Carbs(g) | Fiber (g) | Net Carbs(g) | Protein (g) | Fat (g) |
|---|---|---|---|---|---|---|---|
| Garlic bread, ¾" thick | 1 slice | 150 | 16 | 1 | 15 | 3 | 8 |
| Italian bread | 1 slice | 65 | 12 | 1 | 11 | 2 | 1 |
| Multigrain bread | 1 slice | 65 | 12 | 2 | 10 | 3 | 1 |
| Oat/Oatmeal bread | 1 slice | 73 | 13 | 1 | 12 | 2 | 1 |
| Pita bread, 4" dia | 1 whole | 77 | 16 | 1 | 15 | 3 | Tr |
| Pita bread, 6 ½" dia | 1 whole | 165 | 33 | 1 | 32 | 5 | 1 |
| Potato bread | 1 slice | 100 | 18 | 2 | 16 | 3 | 2 |
| Pumpernickel bread | 1 slice | 80 | 15 | 2 | 13 | 3 | 1 |
| Raisin bread | 1 slice | 100 | 19 | 2 | 17 | 3 | 1 |
| Reduced calorie bread | 1 slice | 45 | 10 | 2 | 8 | 2 | Tr |
| Roll, cinnamon, w/glaze, 3" dia | 1 roll | 200 | 33 | 1 | 32 | 4 | 7 |
| Roll, hard or kaiser | 1 roll | 170 | 30 | 1 | 29 | 6 | 2 |
| Roll, soft, avg size, 1.4 oz | 1 roll | 100 | 18 | 2 | 16 | 2 | 1 |
| Rye bread | 1 slice | 75 | 14 | 2 | 12 | 3 | 1 |
| Sourdough bread | 1 slice | 70 | 13 | 1 | 12 | 2 | 1 |
| Submarine roll, 7" | 1 | 200 | 36 | 4 | 32 | 6 | 4 |
| Vienna bread | 1 slice | 70 | 13 | 1 | 12 | 2 | 1 |
| Wheat bread | 1 slice | 65 | 12 | 1 | 11 | 2 | 1 |
| White bread | 1 slice | 65 | 12 | 1 | 11 | 2 | 1 |
| White or Wheat, light bread | 1 slice | 45 | 10 | 2 | 8 | 2 | Tr |
| (also see Bagel & Biscuit) | | | | | | | |
| **Bread Crumbs** | | | | | | | |
| Dry, grated | 1 cup | 430 | 78 | 3 | 75 | 14 | 6 |
| Dry, seasoned, grated | 1 cup | 440 | 84 | 5 | 79 | 17 | 3 |
| Soft crumbs | 1 cup | 120 | 22 | 2 | 20 | 4 | 2 |
| **Bread Stick** | | | | | | | |
| Crunchy w/ sesame seeds, 0.4 oz | 1 | 40 | 7 | 1 | 6 | 1 | 1 |
| Soft, pizza flavored, 1.5 oz | 1 | 130 | 20 | 1 | 19 | 3 | 4 |
| **Bread Stuffing –** | ... | ... | · | · | · | · | · |
| see Stuffing or Bread Crumbs | | | | | | | |
| **Breakfast Sandwich,** | | | | | | | |
| Biscuit w/ Bacon | 1 | 360 | 27 | 1 | 26 | 9 | 4 |
| Biscuit w/ Egg & Sausage | 1 | 540 | 32 | 1 | 31 | 19 | 37 |
| Biscuit w/ Ham | 1 | 330 | 28 | 1 | 27 | 12 | 20 |
| Biscuit w/ Sausage | 1 | 460 | 28 | 1 | 27 | 12 | 33 |

| | Serving Size | Calories (g) | Total Carbs(g) | Fiber (g) | Net Carbs(g) | Protein (g) | Fat (g) |
|---|---|---|---|---|---|---|---|
| *"Bkfst Sandwich, cont'd"* | | | | | | | |
| Croissant w/Egg, Bacon and Cheese | 1 | 415 | 24 | 2 | 22 | 16 | 28 |
| Croissant w/ Sausage | 1 | 440 | 29 | 2 | 27 | 13 | 32 |
| English Muffin w/ Bacon, Egg, & Cheese | 1 | 370 | 19 | 2 | 17 | 15 | 28 |
| English Muffin w/ Egg, Cheese, & Canadian Bacon | 1 | 290 | 27 | 2 | 25 | 17 | 13 |
| **Broccoli** | | | | | | | |
| *Fresh, raw, flowerets* | *3* | *9* | *3* | *1* | *2* | *Tr* | *Tr* |
| *Fresh, raw, spear, 5" long* | *1* | *9* | *2* | *1* | *1* | *1* | *Tr* |
| *Fresh, raw, chopped or diced* | *1 cup* | *25* | *5* | *3* | *2* | *3* | *Tr* |
| *Fresh, cooked, spear, 5" long* | *1* | *10* | *2* | *1* | *1* | *1* | *Tr* |
| *Fresh, chopped, cooked* | *1 cup* | *44* | *8* | *5* | *3* | *5* | *1* |
| *Frozen, flowerets & cuts, cooked* | *1 cup* | *52* | *10* | *6* | *4* | *6* | *Tr* |
| *Prep w/ butter sauce* | *½ cup* | *75* | *6* | *3* | *3* | *2* | *5* |
| **Broccoli & Rice Casserole** | ¾ cup | 240 | 26 | 5 | 21 | 5 | 12 |
| **Broccoli Au gratin** | ½ cup | 100 | 10 | 3 | 7 | 5 | 4 |
| Broth – see Soup | ... | ... | . | . | . | . | . |
| **Brownie, 2" square** | | | | | | | |
| w/ frosting | 1 square | 190 | 27 | 1 | 26 | 2 | 8 |
| w/o frosting | 1 square | 140 | 20 | 1 | 19 | 2 | 6 |
| Fat Free | 1 square | 90 | 22 | 1 | 21 | 1 | Tr |
| **Brussels Sprouts** | | | | | | | |
| Fresh, cooked | 1 cup | 61 | 14 | 4 | 10 | 4 | 1 |
| Frozen, cooked | 1 cup | 65 | 13 | 6 | 7 | 6 | 1 |
| Prep w/ butter | ½ cup | 75 | 8 | 3 | 5 | 3 | 3 |
| *Bugles* (snacks) | | | | | | | |
| Regular | 1 ¼ cup | 150 | 20 | 1 | 19 | 1 | 7 |
| Baked | 1 ¼ cup | 130 | 23 | 1 | 22 | 2 | 4 |
| Nacho | 1 ¼ cup | 160 | 18 | 1 | 17 | 2 | 9 |
| Ranch | 1 ¼ cup | 160 | 18 | 1 | 17 | 2 | 9 |
| Sour cream & onion | 1 ¼ cup | 160 | 20 | 1 | 19 | 2 | 9 |

| | Serving Size | Calories (g) | Total Carbs(g) | Fiber (g) | Net Carbs(g) | Protein (g) | Fat (g) |
|---|---|---|---|---|---|---|---|
| **Bulgur** | | | | | | | |
| Cooked | 1 cup | 150 | 34 | 8 | 26 | 6 | Tr |
| Uncooked | 1 cup | 480 | 106 | 26 | 80 | 17 | 2 |
| **Bun** – see Bread | ... | ... | . | . | . | . | . |
| **Burrito** | | | | | | | |
| Bean & cheese | 1 | 275 | 25 | 2 | 23 | 10 | 15 |
| Bean & green chili | 1 | 270 | 35 | 3 | 32 | 10 | 9 |
| Beans & rice | 1 | 200 | 36 | 2 | 34 | 6 | 3 |
| Beef & bean | 1 | 300 | 26 | 2 | 24 | 11 | 17 |
| Beef & cheese | 1 | 300 | 26 | 2 | 24 | 10 | 18 |
| Chicken | 1 | 260 | 28 | 2 | 26 | 7 | 10 |
| **Butter** (also see margarine) | | | | | | | |
| **Regular stick,** | | | | | | | |
| **4 sticks/pound** | **1 stick** | **815** | **Tr** | **0** | **Tr** | **1** | **92** |
| **Regular,** | | | | | | | |
| **salted or unsalted** | **1 Tbsp** | **100** | **Tr** | **0** | **Tr** | **Tr** | **12** |
| **Regular,** | | | | | | | |
| **salted or unsalted** | **1 tsp** | **34** | **Tr** | **0** | **Tr** | **Tr** | **4** |
| Apple Butter | 1 Tbsp | 30 | 7 | Tr | 7 | Tr | 0 |
| **Cabbage** | | | | | | | |
| **Green, raw, shredded** | **1 cup** | **18** | **4** | **2** | **2** | **1** | **Tr** |
| **Green, chopped, cooked** | **1 cup** | **33** | **7** | **4** | **3** | **2** | **1** |
| **Chinese cabbage (bok choy)** | | | | | | | |
| **shredded, raw** | **1 cup** | **10** | **2** | **2** | **Tr** | **1** | **Tr** |
| **shredded, cooked** | **1 cup** | **20** | **3** | **3** | **Tr** | **3** | **Tr** |
| **Red cabbage, raw,** | | | | | | | |
| **shredded** | **1 cup** | **19** | **4** | **1** | **3** | **1** | **Tr** |
| **Savoy cabbage, raw,** | | | | | | | |
| **shredded** | **1 cup** | **19** | **4** | **2** | **2** | **1** | **Tr** |
| **Cabbage, Stuffed** | | | | | | | |
| w/ beef or pork | 1 avg | 100 | 9 | 2 | 7 | 6 | 3 |
| **CAKE** (average size slice of single layer cake, 1/8 of 9", unless noted) | | | | | | | |
| Angelfood cake, w/o frosting, | 1 piece | 125 | 28 | Tr | 28 | 3 | Tr |
| Boston Cream Cake | 1 piece | 230 | 39 | 1 | 38 | 2 | 8 |

| | Serving Size | Calories (g) | Total Carbs(g) | Fiber (g) | Net Carbs(g) | Protein (g) | Fat (g) |
|---|---|---|---|---|---|---|---|
| Carrot Cake, | | | | | | | |
| cream cheese icing | 1 piece | 485 | 52 | 2 | 50 | 5 | 29 |
| Cheesecake, | | | | | | | |
| 1/6 of 17 oz cake | 1 piece | 260 | 20 | Tr | 20 | 5 | 18 |
| Cheesecake | | | | | | | |
| w/chocolate, Lg slice | 1 piece | 580 | 44 | 1 | 43 | 9 | 41 |
| Chocolate cake | | | | | | | |
| w/frosting | 1 piece | 390 | 70 | 2 | 68 | 5 | 13 |
| w/o frosting | 1 piece | 290 | 44 | 2 | 42 | 5 | 11 |
| Coffee crumb cake, | | | | | | | |
| 2.2 oz | 1 piece | 265 | 29 | 1 | 28 | 4 | 15 |
| Cupcake – see Cupcakes | ... | ... | . | . | . | . | . |
| Devil's Food cake | | | | | | | |
| w/frosting | 1 piece | 395 | 71 | 2 | 69 | 5 | 13 |
| Fat-free cake, | | | | | | | |
| Chocolate or Vanilla | | | | | | | |
| w/o frosting | 1 piece | 80 | 17 | Tr | 17 | 2 | Tr |
| w/sugar free glaze | 1 piece | 85 | 18 | Tr | 18 | 2 | Tr |
| Fruitcake, small slice | 1 piece | 160 | 27 | 2 | 25 | 1 | 5 |
| Gingerbread | 1 piece | 265 | 36 | 1 | 35 | 3 | 12 |
| Hummingbird | 1 piece | 595 | 72 | 1 | 71 | 5 | 30 |
| Marble cake, w/o frosting | 1 piece | 255 | 34 | 1 | 33 | 3 | 12 |
| Pineapple upside | | | | | | | |
| down cake | 1 piece | 365 | 58 | 1 | 57 | 4 | 14 |
| Pound cake w/o glaze | 1 piece | 220 | 29 | Tr | 29 | 3 | 11 |
| Shortcake, 3" dia | 1 piece | 225 | 32 | 1 | 31 | 4 | 9 |
| Sponge cake | 1 piece | 180 | 35 | Tr | 35 | 5 | 3 |
| White cake, | | | | | | | |
| w/frosting | 1 piece | 395 | 71 | 1 | 70 | 5 | 12 |
| w/o frosting | 1 piece | 265 | 42 | 1 | 41 | 4 | 9 |
| Yellow cake, | | | | | | | |
| w/frosting | 1 piece | 390 | 70 | 1 | 70 | 5 | 12 |
| w/o frosting | 1 piece | 260 | 42 | 1 | 41 | 4 | 9 |
| **CANDY** | | | | | | | |
| *Atomic FireBall*, 3/4" dia | 1 | 24 | 6 | 0 | 6 | 0 | 0 |
| *Almond Joy*, 1.7 oz bar | 1 bar | 240 | 29 | 2 | 27 | 2 | 13 |
| *Baby Ruth*, 2.1 oz bar | 1 bar | 290 | 39 | 1 | 38 | 5 | 13 |
| *Bit-O-Honey*, 2.1 oz | 1 bar | 185 | 39 | Tr | 39 | 1 | 4 |
| **BreathSavers, sugar-free** | **1** | **5** | **2** | **0** | **2** | **0** | **0** |

| | Serving Size | Calories (g) | Total Carbs(g) | Fiber (g) | Net Carbs(g) | Protein (g) | Fat (g) |
|---|---|---|---|---|---|---|---|
| *Butterfinger,* 2.1 oz bar | 1 bar | 280 | 41 | 2 | 39 | 8 | 8 |
| Candy cane, 0.5 oz | 1 cane | 55 | 14 | 0 | 14 | 0 | 0 |
| Candy corn | ¼ cup | 180 | 45 | 0 | 45 | 0 | 1 |
| Caramel | | | | | | | |
| regular caramel, 0.3 oz | 1 piece | 35 | 7 | Tr | 7 | Tr | 1 |
| regular caramel, 2.5 oz | 2.5 oz | 270 | 55 | 1 | 54 | 3 | 6 |
| chocolate | | | | | | | |
| caramel, 0.3 oz | 1 piece | 25 | 6 | Tr | 6 | Tr | Tr |
| Carob | 1 oz | 155 | 16 | 1 | 15 | 2 | 9 |
| Charms Blow Pop | 1 | 60 | 14 | 0 | 14 | 0 | 0 |
| Chocolate Bars | | | | | | | |
| *Hershey's Chocolate bar,* | | | | | | | |
| plain, 1.5 oz bar | 1 bar | 230 | 25 | 1 | 24 | 3 | 13 |
| *Hershey's Nugget,* 10g | 1 bar | 52 | 6 | Tr | 6 | 1 | 3 |
| *Hershey's* | | | | | | | |
| *Snack Size,* 17g | 1 bar | 90 | 10 | Tr | 10 | 1 | 5 |
| with almonds, 1.45 oz | 1 bar | 220 | 22 | 3 | 19 | 4 | 14 |
| with crispy rice, 1.55 oz | 1 bar | 230 | 29 | 1 | 28 | 3 | 12 |
| with peanuts, 1.75 oz | 1 bar | 265 | 25 | 2 | 23 | 5 | 17 |
| (see 'Chocolate for Baking' listed separately) | ... | ... | . | . | . | . | . |
| Chocolate coated peanuts | 10 | 205 | 20 | 2 | 18 | 5 | 13 |
| Chocolate coated raisins | 10 | 40 | 7 | 2 | 5 | Tr | 1 |
| Chocolate Kiss, Hershey's | 4 | 102 | 11 | Tr | 11 | 1 | 6 |
| Fifth Avenue bar, 2 oz | 1 bar | 195 | 26 | 1 | 25 | 4 | 8 |
| Fruit leather bar | 1 oz | 95 | 22 | 1 | 21 | Tr | 2 |
| Fruit leather, small roll | 1 roll | 50 | 12 | 1 | 11 | Tr | Tr |
| Fudge, chocolate, 0.6 oz piece | 1 piece | 65 | 13 | 1 | 12 | Tr | 1 |
| Goobers, 1.4 oz | 1 | 200 | 6 | 0 | 6 | 5 | 13 |
| Gum – see Chewing Gum | ... | ... | . | . | . | . | . |
| Gumdrops, ¾" dia | 5 | 64 | 16 | 0 | 16 | 0 | 0 |
| Gummy Bears | 10 | 85 | 22 | 0 | 22 | 0 | 0 |
| Gummy Worms | 10 | 285 | 73 | 0 | 73 | 0 | 0 |
| Hard Candy, regular, 1" dia | | | | | | | |
| Butterscotch or Coffee flavor | 2 | 42 | 10 | 0 | 10 | 0 | 0 |
| Cinnamon, Fruit, or Mint flavor | 2 | 40 | 10 | 0 | 10 | 0 | 0 |

| | Serving Size | Calories (g) | Total Carbs(g) | Fiber (g) | Net Carbs(g) | Protein (g) | Fat (g) |
|---|---|---|---|---|---|---|---|
| Hard Candy, sugar free | | | | | | | |
| Baskin Robbins, sugar-free Fruit or Chocolate Mint | 2 | 20 | 7 | 0 | 7 | 0 | 1 |
| Brachs, sugar-free Cinnamon | 3 | 35 | 17 | 0 | 17 | 0 | 0 |
| Life Savers, sugar-free | 4 | 30 | 14 | 0 | 14 | 0 | 0 |
| Sweet 'N Low Fruit Flavors | 5 | 30 | 14 | 0 | 14 | 0 | 0 |
| Sweet 'N Low Butterscotch | 5 | 30 | 15 | 0 | 15 | 0 | 0 |
| Sweet 'N Low Coffee | 5 | 30 | 14 | 0 | 14 | 0 | 0 |
| Jawbreaker, regular size, ³/₄" dia | 1 | 24 | 6 | 0 | 6 | 0 | 0 |
| Jawbreaker, large size, 1" dia | 1 | 40 | 9 | 0 | 9 | 0 | 0 |
| Jelly Beans, regular size | 10 | 100 | 25 | 0 | 25 | 0 | Tr |
| Jelly Beans, small pieces | 10 | 40 | 10 | 0 | 10 | 0 | Tr |
| Kit Kat bar, 1.5 oz | 1 bar | 215 | 27 | Tr | 27 | 3 | 11 |
| Krackel bar, 1.5 oz | 1 bar | 220 | 25 | 1 | 24 | 3 | 12 |
| Licorice, 1.4 oz pkg | 1.4 oz | 135 | 31 | 0 | 31 | 1 | 1 |
| LifeSavers | 2 | 20 | 5 | 0 | 5 | 0 | 0 |
| Lollipop, Charms Blow Pop, 15g | 1 | 60 | 14 | 0 | 14 | 0 | 0 |
| Lollipop, large, 14 g | 1 | 50 | 12 | 0 | 12 | 0 | 0 |
| Lollipop, small, Dum Dum, 5 g | 1 | 24 | 6 | 0 | 6 | 0 | 0 |
| M&M candy, plain | 10 | 34 | 5 | Tr | 5 | Tr | 1 |
| M&M candy, w/ nuts | 10 | 103 | 12 | 1 | 11 | 2 | 5 |
| Mars Almond bar, 1.75 oz | 1 bar | 235 | 31 | 2 | 29 | 4 | 12 |
| Marshmallow, avg size | 1 | 23 | 6 | 0 | 6 | 0 | 0 |
| Milky Way, regular size, 2.15 oz | 1 bar | 258 | 44 | 1 | 43 | 3 | 10 |
| Milky Way, small, fun size | 1 bar | 76 | 13 | Tr | 13 | 1 | 3 |
| Mints, pastel, ¹/₂" square | 10 mints | 75 | 18 | 0 | 18 | 0 | 0 |
| Mounds, 1.9 oz bar | 1 bar | 255 | 31 | 2 | 29 | 2 | 13 |
| Mr. Goodbar, 1.75 oz | 1 bar | 265 | 25 | 2 | 23 | 5 | 17 |
| Oh Henry, 2 oz bar | 1 bar | 245 | 37 | 1 | 36 | 6 | 10 |
| Nestle Crunch bar, 1.55 oz | 1 bar | 230 | 29 | 1 | 28 | 3 | 12 |
| Peanut Brittle | 1 oz | 130 | 20 | 1 | 19 | 2 | 5 |
| Peppermint Pattie, 1.5 oz | 1 pattie | 165 | 34 | 1 | 33 | 1 | 3 |

| | Serving Size | Calories (g) | Total Carbs(g) | Fiber (g) | Net Carbs(g) | Protein (g) | Fat (g) |
|---|---|---|---|---|---|---|---|
| *Raisinets*, 1.6 oz pkg | 1 pkg | 185 | 32 | 6 | 26 | 2 | 7 |
| *Reese's Peanut Butter Cups* | | | | | | | |
| regular size cups | 2 cups | 245 | 25 | 1 | 24 | 5 | 14 |
| ***miniature size cups*** | ***2 cups*** | ***42*** | ***4*** | ***Tr*** | ***4*** | ***1*** | ***2*** |
| *Reese's Pieces*, 1.6 oz pkg | 1 pkg | 225 | 28 | 1 | 27 | 6 | 9 |
| *Reese Sticks*, 0.6 oz bar | 1 bar | 90 | 9 | Tr | 9 | 2 | 1 |
| *Rolo caramels* | 9 pieces | 220 | 28 | 1 | 27 | 3 | 11 |
| *Skittles*, 2.3 oz pkg | 1 pkg | 265 | 59 | Tr | 59 | 0 | 3 |
| *Skor toffee bar*, 1.4 oz | 1 bar | 220 | 23 | Tr | 23 | 13 | 2 |
| *Snickers bar,* | | | | | | | |
| regular size, 2 oz | 1 bar | 275 | 34 | 1 | 33 | 5 | 14 |
| *Snickers bar,* | | | | | | | |
| small fun size | 1 bar | 72 | 9 | Tr | 9 | 1 | 4 |
| *Special Dark,* | | | | | | | |
| miniature bar | 1 bar | 46 | 5 | Tr | 5 | Tr | 3 |
| *Starburst Fruit Chews,* | | | | | | | |
| 2 oz pkg | 1 pkg | 235 | 50 | 0 | 50 | Tr | 5 |
| *Starlight Mints,* 1" dia | 3 | 56 | 14 | 0 | 14 | 0 | 0 |
| Sucker – see Lollipop | ... | ... | . | . | . | . | . |
| *Three Musketeers,* | | | | | | | |
| 2.1 oz bar | 1 bar | 250 | 46 | Tr | 46 | 2 | 8 |
| *Toffee,* 1.4 oz bar | 1 bar | 220 | 23 | 1 | 22 | 2 | 13 |
| *Tootsie Roll,* 1 oz | 1 oz | 110 | 15 | Tr | 15 | 1 | 6 |
| *Twizzlers,* Cherry, | | | | | | | |
| 2.5 oz pkg | 1 pkg | 135 | 31 | 0 | 31 | 1 | 1 |
| **Cannelloni, Cheese** | | | | | | | |
| *Lean Cuisine entrée* | 1 meal | 250 | 30 | 2 | 28 | 16 | 6 |
| **Cantaloupe** | | | | | | | |
| Fresh, medium size, | | | | | | | |
| 5" dia | ½ melon | 98 | 22 | 2 | 20 | 3 | Tr |
| Fresh, wedge ⅛ melon | 1 wedge | 25 | 6 | 1 | 5 | 1 | Tr |
| Fresh, cubed | 1 cup | 55 | 13 | 1 | 12 | 1 | Tr |
| **Carambola** (starfruit) | | | | | | | |
| ***Fresh, 3 ½", whole*** | ***1*** | ***30*** | ***7*** | ***3*** | ***4*** | ***Tr*** | ***Tr*** |
| Fresh, sliced | 1 cup | 36 | 8 | 3 | 5 | 1 | Tr |
| **Caramels** – see candy | ... | ... | . | . | . | . | . |
| **Carrot** | | | | | | | |
| Fresh, raw, whole, | | | | | | | |
| 7 ½" long | 1 | 32 | 7 | 2 | 5 | 1 | Tr |

| | Serving Size | Calories (g) | Total Carbs(g) | Fiber (g) | Net Carbs(g) | Protein (g) | Fat (g) |
|---|---|---|---|---|---|---|---|
| Fresh, raw, shredded | 1 cup | 47 | 11 | 3 | 8 | 1 | Tr |
| *Fresh, baby carrots* | *2* | *12* | *3* | *1* | *2* | *Tr* | *Tr* |
| Fresh, cooked, slices | 1 cup | 65 | 14 | 5 | 9 | 2 | Tr |
| Frozen, cooked, slices | 1 cup | 69 | 15 | 5 | 10 | 2 | Tr |
| Canned, drained, slices, cooked | 1 cup | 57 | 13 | 3 | 10 | 1 | Tr |
| Glazed carrots | ³/₄ cup | 280 | 35 | 5 | 30 | 1 | 15 |
| **Cashew** – see Nuts | ... | ... | . | . | . | . | . |
| **Casserole,** see specific listings | ... | ... | . | . | . | . | . |
| ***Catsup, regular*** | *1 Tbsp* | *18* | *4* | *Tr* | *4* | *Tr* | *Tr* |
| ***Restaurant size packet*** | *1 pkt* | *10* | *3* | *Tr* | *3* | *Tr* | *Tr* |
| **Cauliflower** | | | | | | | |
| ***Fresh, raw, flowerets*** | *3* | *9* | *3* | *1* | *2* | *Tr* | *Tr* |
| ***Fresh, raw, chopped or diced*** | *1 cup* | *25* | *5* | *3* | *2* | *2* | *Tr* |
| ***Fresh, flowerets, cooked*** | *3* | *12* | *2* | *1* | *1* | *1* | *Tr* |
| ***Fresh, chopped, cooked*** | *1 cup* | *30* | *5* | *3* | *2* | *2* | *Tr* |
| ***Frozen, cuts, cooked*** | *1 cup* | *35* | *7* | *5* | *2* | *3* | *Tr* |
| ***Prep w/ butter*** | *³/₄ cup* | *100* | *6* | *2* | *4* | *2* | *8* |
| ***Prep w/ cheese sauce*** | *³/₄ cup* | *110* | *6* | *2* | *4* | *4* | *8* |
| Cavatelli | 1 cup | 400 | 77 | 1 | 76 | 14 | 2 |
| **Caviar** – see Fish | ... | ... | . | . | . | . | . |
| ***Cayenne, dried spice*** | *¹/₄ tsp* | *1* | *Tr* | *Tr* | *Tr* | *Tr* | *0* |
| Caesar Salad | 4 oz | 200 | 7 | 2 | 5 | 7 | 17 |
| **Celery** | | | | | | | |
| ***Fresh, raw, stalk, 7 1/2" long*** | *1 stalk* | *6* | *1* | *Tr* | *Tr* | *Tr* | *Tr* |
| ***Fresh, raw, diced*** | *1 cup* | *19* | *4* | *2* | *2* | *1* | *Tr* |
| ***Cooked, stalk 7 1/2" long*** | *1 stalk* | *6* | *1* | *Tr* | *Tr* | *Tr* | *Tr* |
| ***Cooked, diced pieces*** | *1 cup* | *27* | *6* | *2* | *4* | *1* | *Tr* |
| ***Celery Seed*** | *1 tsp* | *8* | *1* | *Tr* | *Tr* | *Tr* | *1* |
| **CEREAL** | | | | | | | |
| *All-Bran* | ¹/₂ cup | 80 | 23 | 10 | 13 | 4 | 1 |
| *Apple Jacks* | 1 cup | 116 | 27 | 1 | 26 | 1 | Tr |
| *Cap'n Crunch, regular* | ³/₄ cup | 107 | 23 | 1 | 22 | 1 | 1 |
| *Crunchberries* | ³/₄ cup | 104 | 22 | 1 | 21 | 1 | 1 |

| | Serving Size | Calories (g) | Total Carbs(g) | Fiber (g) | Net Carbs(g) | Protein (g) | Fat (g) |
|---|---|---|---|---|---|---|---|
| *Peanut Butter Crunchy* | ¾ cup | 112 | 22 | 1 | 21 | 2 | 2 |
| *Cheerios Cereal, regular* | 1 cup | 110 | 23 | 3 | 20 | 3 | 2 |
| Apple Cinnamon Cheerios | ¾ cup | 118 | 25 | 2 | 23 | 2 | 2 |
| *Honey Nut Cheerios* | 1 cup | 115 | 24 | 2 | 22 | 3 | 1 |
| *Chex Cereal, Corn* | 1 cup | 110 | 26 | 1 | 25 | 2 | Tr |
| *Honey Nut* | ¾ cup | 120 | 26 | Tr | 26 | 2 | 1 |
| *Multi Bran* | 1 cup | 200 | 39 | 5 | 34 | 4 | 1 |
| *Rice* | 1 ¼ cup | 120 | 27 | Tr | 27 | 2 | Tr |
| *Wheat* | 1 cup | 180 | 24 | 3 | 21 | 3 | 1 |
| *Cinnamon Toast Crunch* | ¾ cup | 124 | 24 | 2 | 22 | 2 | 3 |
| *Cocoa Krispies* | ¾ cup | 120 | 27 | Tr | 27 | 2 | 1 |
| *Cocoa Puffs* | 1 cup | 120 | 27 | Tr | 27 | 1 | 1 |
| Corn Flakes | 1 cup | 105 | 24 | 1 | 23 | 2 | Tr |
| Corn Pops | 1 cup | 118 | 28 | Tr | 28 | 1 | Tr |
| Cream of Wheat, as prep | 1 cup | 130 | 27 | 1 | 26 | 4 | Tr |
| *Crispix* | 1 cup | 108 | 25 | 1 | 24 | 2 | Tr |
| Fruit Loops | 1 cup | 117 | 26 | 1 | 25 | 1 | 1 |
| Frosted Flakes | 1 cup | 120 | 28 | 1 | 27 | 1 | Tr |
| Frosted Mini Wheats | | | | | | | |
| regular size | 1 cup | 175 | 42 | 6 | 36 | 5 | 1 |
| bite size | 1 cup | 190 | 45 | 6 | 39 | 5 | 1 |
| *Golden Grahams* | ¾ cup | 116 | 26 | 1 | 25 | 2 | 1 |
| Granola Cereal, | | | | | | | |
| *Nature Valley* | ¾ cup | 250 | 36 | 4 | 32 | 6 | 10 |
| *Kix Cereal, regular* | 1 ¼ cup | 114 | 26 | 1 | 25 | 2 | 1 |
| *Kix Berry Berry* | ¾ cup | 120 | 26 | Tr | 26 | 1 | 1 |
| *Life, regular* | ¾ cup | 120 | 25 | 2 | 23 | 3 | 1 |
| *Life Cinnamon* | 1 cup | 190 | 40 | 3 | 37 | 4 | 2 |
| *Lucky Charms* | 1 cup | 116 | 25 | 1 | 24 | 2 | 1 |
| *Malt O Meal*, as prep | 1 cup | 122 | 26 | 1 | 25 | 4 | Tr |
| Oat Cereal, Cheerios type | 1 cup | 110 | 23 | 3 | 20 | 3 | 2 |
| Oatmeal, warm | ... | ... | · | · | · | · | · |
| – see Oatmeal | | | | | | | |
| Peanut Butter | | | | | | | |
| Puffed Cereal | ¾ cup | 130 | 23 | Tr | 23 | 3 | 3 |
| *Product 19* | 1 cup | 110 | 25 | 1 | 24 | 3 | Tr |
| Puffed Rice | 1 cup | 56 | 13 | Tr | 13 | 1 | Tr |
| Puffed Wheat | 1 cup | 44 | 10 | 1 | 9 | 2 | Tr |
| Raisin Bran | 1 cup | 180 | 45 | 7 | 38 | 1 | 1 |
| Raisin Nut Bran | 1 cup | 210 | 41 | 5 | 36 | 5 | 4 |

| | Serving Size | Calories (g) | Total Carbs(g) | Fiber (g) | Net Carbs(g) | Protein (g) | Fat (g) |
|---|---|---|---|---|---|---|---|
| Rice Crispies | 1 ¼ cup | 124 | 29 | Tr | 29 | 2 | Tr |
| Shredded Wheat, | | | | | | | |
| large frosted biscuits | 2 biscuits | 155 | 38 | 5 | 33 | 5 | 1 |
| *Smacks* | ¾ cup | 105 | 24 | 1 | 23 | 2 | Tr |
| *Special K* | 1 cup | 115 | 22 | 1 | 21 | 6 | Tr |
| *Total* | ¾ cup | 105 | 24 | 3 | 21 | 3 | 1 |
| *Trix* | 1 cup | 122 | 26 | 1 | 25 | 1 | 2 |
| Wheat Bran Flakes | ¾ cup | 95 | 23 | 5 | 18 | 3 | 1 |
| *Wheaties* | 1 cup | 110 | 24 | 2 | 22 | 3 | 1 |
| **Cereal Bar** | | | | | | | |
| Plain | 1 bar | 135 | 28 | 1 | 27 | 2 | 2 |
| Fruit filled | 1 bar | 145 | 29 | 1 | 28 | 2 | 2 |
| **Chalupa** | | | | | | | |
| Beef | 1 | 380 | 29 | 2 | 27 | 14 | 23 |
| Chicken | 1 | 360 | 28 | 2 | 26 | 17 | 20 |
| Nacho cheese & beef | 1 | 370 | 30 | 2 | 28 | 13 | 22 |
| Nacho cheese & chicken | 1 | 350 | 29 | 2 | 27 | 16 | 19 |
| Nacho cheese & steak | 1 | 350 | 28 | 2 | 26 | 16 | 19 |
| **CHEESE** | | | | | | | |
| American, | | | | | | | |
| pasteurized cheese | | | | | | | |
| **regular** | **1 oz** | **105** | **1** | **0** | **1** | **6** | **9** |
| **fat free** | **1 slice** | **25** | **3** | **0** | **3** | **4** | **0** |
| **Blue cheese** | **1 oz** | **100** | **1** | **0** | **1** | **6** | **8** |
| **Camembert, 1.3 oz** | **1 wedge** | **114** | **Tr** | **0** | **Tr** | **8** | **9** |
| Cheddar cheese regular, | | | | | | | |
| **1 oz slice** | **1 slice** | **115** | **Tr** | **0** | **Tr** | **7** | **9** |
| **1" cube** | **1 cube** | **68** | **Tr** | **0** | **Tr** | **4** | **6** |
| **shredded** | **1 cup** | **455** | **1** | **0** | **1** | **28** | **37** |
| **lowfat** | **1 oz** | **50** | **1** | **0** | **1** | **7** | **2** |
| **fat free** | **1 slice** | **25** | **3** | **0** | **3** | **4** | **0** |
| **Cheese food,** | | | | | | | |
| **pasteurized** | **1 oz** | **93** | **2** | **0** | **2** | **6** | **7** |
| **Cheese spread,** | | | | | | | |
| **pasteurized** | **1 oz** | **82** | **2** | **0** | **2** | **5** | **6** |
| **Colby cheese** | **1 oz** | **112** | **1** | **0** | **1** | **7** | **9** |
| Cottage cheese | | | | | | | |
| regular, creamed, 4% fat | | | | | | | |
| large curd | 1 cup | 233 | 6 | 0 | 6 | 28 | 10 |
| small curd | 1 cup | 217 | 6 | 0 | 6 | 26 | 9 |

| | Serving Size | Calories (g) | Total Carbs(g) | Fiber (g) | Net Carbs(g) | Protein (g) | Fat (g) |
|---|---|---|---|---|---|---|---|
| with fruit | 1 cup | 279 | 30 | 0 | 30 | 22 | 8 |
| lowfat, 2% fat | 1 cup | 203 | 8 | 0 | 8 | 31 | 4 |
| lowfat, 1% fat | 1 cup | 164 | 6 | 0 | 6 | 28 | 2 |
| fat free | 1 cup | 160 | 10 | 0 | 10 | 30 | 0 |
| **dry curd, uncreamed, 0.5% fat** | **1 cup** | **123** | **3** | **0** | **3** | **25** | **1** |
| Cream cheese | | | | | | | |
| **regular cream** | **1 oz** | **100** | **1** | **0** | **1** | **2** | **10** |
| **regular cream** | **1 Tbsp** | **50** | **Tr** | **0** | **Tr** | **1** | **5** |
| **lowfat/light** | **1 Tbsp** | **35** | **1** | **0** | **1** | **2** | **3** |
| **fat free** | **1 Tbsp** | **15** | **1** | **0** | **1** | **2** | **0** |
| **Feta** | **1 oz** | **75** | **1** | **0** | **1** | **4** | **6** |
| **Fontina** | **1 oz** | **110** | **1** | **0** | **1** | **7** | **9** |
| **Goat cheese, soft** | **1 oz** | **75** | **1** | **0** | **1** | **4** | **6** |
| **Monterey jack, processed** | **1 oz** | **105** | **Tr** | **0** | **Tr** | **7** | **9** |
| **Jalapeno jack, processed** | **1 oz** | **90** | **1** | **0** | **1** | **5** | **8** |
| **Mozzarella** | | | | | | | |
| **regular, 1 oz slice** | **1 slice** | **80** | **1** | **0** | **1** | **8** | **5** |
| **shredded, 2 oz** | **½ cup** | **160** | **2** | **0** | **2** | **16** | **10** |
| **fat free** | **1 slice** | **25** | **3** | **0** | **3** | **4** | **0** |
| **Muenster, sliced** | **1 oz** | **105** | **Tr** | **0** | **Tr** | **7** | **9** |
| **Neufchatel** | **1 oz** | **75** | **1** | **0** | **1** | **3** | **7** |
| **Parmesan** | | | | | | | |
| **grated** | **1 cup** | **455** | **4** | **0** | **4** | **42** | **30** |
| **grated** | **1 Tbsp** | **25** | **Tr** | **0** | **Tr** | **2** | **2** |
| **Provolone** | **1 oz** | **100** | **1** | **0** | **1** | **7** | **8** |
| Ricotta cheese | | | | | | | |
| regular | 1 cup | 430 | 7 | 0 | 7 | 28 | 32 |
| part skim | 1 cup | 340 | 13 | 0 | 13 | 28 | 19 |
| fat free | 1 cup | 240 | 20 | 0 | 20 | 40 | 0 |
| **Romano, grated** | **1 oz** | **110** | **1** | **0** | **1** | **9** | **8** |
| **Roquefort, sheep's milk** | **1 oz** | **105** | **1** | **0** | **1** | **6** | **9** |
| Swiss | | | | | | | |
| **regular, 1 oz slice** | **1 slice** | **105** | **1** | **0** | **1** | **8** | **8** |
| **fat free** | **1 slice** | **25** | **3** | **0** | **3** | **4** | **0** |
| Cheese Puffs (about 25) | 1 oz | 160 | 15 | Tr | 15 | 2 | 10 |
| Cheese Puffs Balls (2 ½ cups) | 1 oz | 160 | 15 | Tr | 15 | 2 | 10 |

| | Serving Size | Calories (g) | Total Carbs (g) | Fiber (g) | Net Carbs (g) | Protein (g) | Fat (g) |
|---|---|---|---|---|---|---|---|
| **Cheese Spread** | | | | | | | |
| **Cheez Whiz** | **2 Tbsp** | **90** | **2** | **0** | **2** | **5** | **7** |
| **Velveeta** | **2 Tbsp** | **80** | **3** | **0** | **3** | **5** | **6** |
| **Cheetos** (snacks) | | | | | | | |
| Curls (about 15) | 1 oz | 150 | 15 | Tr | 15 | 2 | 10 |
| Puffs (about 25) | 1 oz | 160 | 15 | Tr | 15 | 2 | 10 |
| **Cherries** | | | | | | | |
| Fresh, sweet | 10 | 50 | 11 | 2 | 9 | 1 | 1 |
| Sour, canned, water pack | 1 cup | 90 | 22 | 3 | 19 | 2 | Tr |
| **Cherry Pie Filling**, canned | 3 oz | 80 | 20 | Tr | 20 | Tr | Tr |
| **Chestnut** – see Nuts | ... | ... | . | . | . | . | . |
| **Chewing Gum** | | | | | | | |
| Stick Gum, | | | | | | | |
| 2 ¾" long, all flavors | | | | | | | |
| **Wrigley's, regular** | **1 stick** | **10** | **2** | **0** | **2** | **0** | **0** |
| **Wrigley's Extra,** | | | | | | | |
| **sugar-free** | **1 stick** | **5** | **2** | **0** | **2** | **0** | **0** |
| **Carefree, sugar-free** | **1 stick** | **5** | **2** | **0** | **2** | **0** | **0** |
| Bubble Yum, | | | | | | | |
| all regular flavors | 1 | 25 | 6 | 0 | 6 | 0 | 0 |
| **Dentyne Ice, all flavors** | **2** | **5** | **2** | **0** | **2** | **0** | **0** |
| Gum Balls, | | | | | | | |
| small, ½" dia balls | 5 | 40 | 10 | 0 | 10 | 0 | 0 |
| Gum Balls, | | | | | | | |
| Lg, 1 ¼" dia balls | 1 | 32 | 8 | 0 | 8 | 0 | 0 |
| **Grapermelon,** | | | | | | | |
| **Wrigley's, ¾"** | **2** | **10** | **2** | **0** | **2** | **0** | **0** |
| **Strappleberry,** | | | | | | | |
| **Wrigley's , ¾"** | **2** | **10** | **2** | **0** | **2** | **0** | **0** |
| **Trident, all flavors,** | | | | | | | |
| **1" sticks** | **1 stick** | **5** | **1** | **0** | **1** | **0** | **0** |
| Chex Mix, 1 oz | ⅔ cup | 120 | 18 | 2 | 16 | 3 | 5 |
| **CHICKEN** | | | | | | | |
| **Giblets, simmered,** | | | | | | | |
| **chopped** | **1 cup** | **230** | **1** | **0** | **1** | **37** | **7** |
| Fried Chicken, | | | | | | | |
| batter dipped | | | | | | | |
| ½ breast, about | | | | | | | |
| 5 oz meat | 1 | 365 | 13 | Tr | 13 | 35 | 18 |

| | Serving Size | Calories (g) | Total Carbs(g) | Fiber (g) | Net Carbs(g) | Protein (g) | Fat (g) |
|---|---|---|---|---|---|---|---|
| Drumstick, avg size | 1 | 195 | 6 | Tr | 6 | 16 | 11 |
| Thigh, avg size | 1 | 240 | 8 | Tr | 8 | 19 | 14 |
| Wing, avg size | 1 | 160 | 5 | Tr | 5 | 10 | 11 |
| Strips, dark meat | 3 oz | 205 | 10 | Tr | 10 | 25 | 9 |
| Strips, white meat | 3 oz | 175 | 7 | Tr | 7 | 25 | 5 |
| *Liver of chicken, simmered* | *1* | *31* | *Tr* | *0* | *Tr* | *5* | *1* |
| *Neck, simmered* | *1* | *32* | *0* | *0* | *0* | *4* | *1* |
| Roasted or Broiled Chicken | | | | | | | |
| *½ Breast, about 3.5 oz meat* | *½ breast* | *165* | *0* | *0* | *0* | *32* | *4* |
| *Drumstick, avg size* | *1* | *75* | *0* | *0* | *0* | *12* | *2* |
| *Thigh, avg size* | *1* | *110* | *0* | *0* | *0* | *13* | *6* |
| *White meat w/ skin* | *3.5 oz* | *280* | *0* | *0* | *0* | *33* | *12* |
| *White meat, skinless* | *3.5 oz* | *170* | *0* | *0* | *0* | *33* | *4* |
| *Dark meat w/ skin* | *3.5 oz* | *320* | *0* | *0* | *0* | *22* | *21* |
| *Dark meat skinless* | *3.5 oz* | *190* | *0* | *0* | *0* | *22* | *10* |
| *Canned, boneless* | *5 oz* | *235* | *0* | *0* | *0* | *31* | *11* |
| Stewed Chicken | | | | | | | |
| *Light & dark meat, diced* | *1 cup* | *330* | *0* | *0* | *0* | *43* | *17* |
| *Wings, Buffalo, hot* | *3* | *210* | *3* | *0* | *3* | *22* | *12* |
| *Wings, Buffalo, mild* | *4* | *200* | *0* | *0* | *0* | *23* | *12* |
| (Other Chicken Products, see: Bologna, Hot Dog, Salami, Sausage & specific entrées) | ... | ... | . | . | . | . | . |
| **Chicken a la King** | 1 cup | 320 | 17 | Tr | 17 | 15 | 22 |
| **Chicken Alfredo** | 1 cup | 300 | 35 | Tr | 35 | 18 | 10 |
| Chicken & Broccoli Alfredo | 1½ cups | 300 | 38 | 1 | 37 | 25 | 6 |
| **Chicken Cacciatoré** | | | | | | | |
| *Healthy Choice entrée* | 1 meal | 250 | 36 | 1 | 35 | 21 | 3 |
| *Lean Cuisine entrée* | 1 meal | 280 | 25 | 1 | 24 | 23 | 10 |
| **Chicken Cordon Blue** | | | | | | | |
| *Le Menu entrée* | 1 meal | 460 | 48 | 1 | 47 | 23 | 20 |
| **Chicken Dijon,** | | | | | | | |
| *Healthy Choice* | 1 meal | 270 | 33 | 1 | 32 | 23 | 5 |

| | Serving Size | Calories (g) | Total Carbs(g) | Fiber (g) | Net Carbs(g) | Protein (g) | Fat (g) |
|---|---|---|---|---|---|---|---|
| **Chicken Francesca** | | | | | | | |
| *Healthy Choice entrée* | 1 meal | 330 | 46 | 1 | 45 | 23 | 6 |
| **Chicken Kiev,** | | | | | | | |
| *Tyson entrée* | 1 meal | 440 | 36 | 1 | 35 | 18 | 25 |
| **Chicken Marsala,** | | | | | | | |
| *Tyson entrée* | 1 meal | 180 | 19 | 1 | 18 | 15 | 5 |
| **Chicken Nuggets** | | | | | | | |
| *Banquet entrée* | 1 meal | 410 | 38 | 1 | 37 | 18 | 21 |
| *Morton entrée* | 1 meal | 320 | 30 | 1 | 29 | 13 | 17 |
| **Chicken Parmagiana** | | | | | | | |
| *Banquet entrée* | 1 meal | 290 | 27 | 1 | 26 | 14 | 15 |
| *Healthy Choice entrée* | 1 meal | 300 | 47 | 1 | 46 | 20 | 4 |
| *Le Menu entrée* | 1 meal | 395 | 30 | 1 | 29 | 26 | 19 |
| ***Chicken Roll, light meat*** | ***2 oz*** | ***90*** | ***2*** | ***1*** | ***1*** | ***11*** | ***4*** |
| **Chicken Teriyaki** | | | | | | | |
| w/vegetables | 1 cup | 200 | 20 | 2 | 18 | 12 | 8 |
| **Chicken w/Sweet** | | | | | | | |
| **& Sour Sauce** | 1 cup | 320 | 53 | 2 | 51 | 19 | 5 |
| **Chicken w/Vegetables** | | | | | | | |
| *Lean Cuisine entrée* | 1 meal | 250 | 33 | 2 | 31 | 18 | 5 |
| **Chickpeas,** cooked | ½ cup | 140 | 25 | 6 | 19 | 7 | 2 |
| ***Chili Powder*** | ***1 tsp*** | ***8*** | ***1*** | ***Tr*** | ***Tr*** | ***Tr*** | ***Tr*** |
| **Chili w/Beans** | 1 cup | 270 | 23 | 8 | 15 | 21 | 11 |
| Con Carne w/Beans | 1 cup | 255 | 24 | 8 | 16 | 20 | 8 |
| **Chimichanga** | | | | | | | |
| Beans & cheese | 1 | 300 | 25 | 1 | 24 | 9 | 17 |
| Beef & cheese | 1 | 425 | 43 | 1 | 42 | 20 | 20 |
| Chicken & cheese | 1 | 350 | 39 | 1 | 38 | 11 | 16 |
| **Chips** – see other specific listings | | | | | | | |
| ***Chives, raw, chopped*** | ***1 Tbsp*** | ***1*** | ***Tr*** | ***Tr*** | ***Tr*** | ***Tr*** | ***Tr*** |
| **Chocolate for Baking** (Also see 'Candy' for other chocolates) | | | | | | | |
| Chocolate Chips, milk, regular | 1 cup | 860 | 99 | 6 | 93 | 12 | 52 |

| | Serving Size | Calories (g) | Total Carbs(g) | Fiber (g) | Net Carbs(g) | Protein (g) | Fat (g) |
|---|---|---|---|---|---|---|---|
| Chocolate Chips, semisweet | 1 cup | 805 | 106 | 10 | 96 | 7 | 50 |
| Chocolate Chips, white | 1 cup | 915 | 101 | 0 | 101 | 10 | 55 |
| ***Unsweetened for baking, solid*** | *1 square* | *148* | *8* | *4* | *4* | *3* | *16* |
| Unsweetened, liquid | 1 oz | 134 | 10 | 5 | 5 | 3 | 14 |
| **Chow Mein** | | | | | | | |
| Beef chow mein | 1 ½ cups | 170 | 12 | 2 | 10 | 14 | 6 |
| Chicken chow mein | 1 ½ cups | 160 | 12 | 2 | 10 | 14 | 7 |
| ***Cilantro, raw*** | *1 tsp* | *Tr* | *Tr* | *Tr* | *Tr* | *Tr* | *Tr* |
| ***Cinnamon*** | *1 tsp* | *6* | *2* | *1* | *1* | *Tr* | *Tr* |
| **Cinnamon Sweet Roll** | | | | | | | |
| w/ glaze, 3" dia | 1 | 200 | 33 | 1 | 32 | 4 | 7 |
| w/ raisins & glaze, 3" dia | 1 | 225 | 35 | 1 | 34 | 4 | 10 |
| w/ raisins & glaze, 4 ½" dia | 1 | 510 | 85 | 2 | 83 | 8 | 15 |
| **Clam Chowder** – see Soup | ... | ... | . | . | | . | . |
| **Clams** – see Fish/Seafood | ... | ... | . | . | . | . | . |
| ***Cloves, ground*** | *1 tsp* | *6* | *1* | *Tr* | *Tr* | *Tr* | *Tr* |
| ***Cocoa, unsweetened powder*** | *1 Tbsp* | *15* | *3* | *2* | *1* | *1* | *1* |
| | 1 cup | 240 | 48 | 32 | 16 | 16 | 16 |
| Coconut | | | | | | | |
| ***Fresh piece, 2" x 2" x ½"*** | *1 piece* | *160* | *7* | *4* | *3* | *1* | *15* |
| Fresh, shredded, not packed | 1 cup | 285 | 12 | 7 | 5 | 3 | 27 |
| Dried, sweetened, flaked | 1 cup | 465 | 44 | 4 | 40 | 3 | 33 |
| Coleslaw | ½ cup | 62 | 10 | 1 | 9 | 1 | 2 |
| Collards | | | | | | | |
| ***Fresh, chopped, cooked*** | *1 cup* | *49* | *9* | *5* | *4* | *4* | *1* |
| Frozen, chopped, cooked | 1 cup | 61 | 12 | 5 | 7 | 5 | 1 |
| **Condiments**, see Sauce, or see specific listing | ... | ... | . | . | | . | . |

| | Serving Size | Calories (g) | Total Carbs(g) | Fiber (g) | Net Carbs(g) | Protein (g) | Fat (g) |
|---|---|---|---|---|---|---|---|
| **COOKIES** | | | | | | | |
| 2 ¼" dia unless noted | | | | | | | |
| Animal Crackers, 1" dia | 8 | 60 | 12 | Tr | 12 | 1 | 1 |
| Butter Cookie | 1 | 50 | 7 | Tr | 7 | Tr | 2 |
| Chocolate Chip, regular | 1 | 80 | 12 | 1 | 11 | 2 | 3 |
| reduced fat | 1 | 70 | 12 | 1 | 11 | 2 | 1 |
| sugar-free | 1 | 70 | 10 | 1 | 9 | 1 | 6 |
| Coconut cookie | 1 | 75 | 11 | 1 | 10 | 1 | 3 |
| Newton | 2 | 110 | 20 | 1 | 19 | 1 | 2 |
| Molasses cookie | 1 | 80 | 13 | Tr | 13 | 1 | 2 |
| Oatmeal w/ raisins | 1 | 75 | 12 | 1 | 11 | 1 | 2 |
| plain | 1 | 70 | 11 | 1 | 10 | 1 | 2 |
| sugar-free | 1 | 70 | 10 | 1 | 9 | 1 | 6 |
| Peanut Butter, plain | 1 | 80 | 10 | Tr | 10 | 1 | 2 |
| w/ nuts | 1 | 90 | 11 | Tr | 11 | 2 | 3 |
| Pecan Shortbread cookie | 1 | 75 | 8 | Tr | 8 | 1 | 5 |
| Sandwich cookie, 1 ½" dia, round, | | | | | | | |
| chocolate w/crème filling | 1 | 50 | 7 | Tr | 7 | Tr | 2 |
| sugar w/ peanut butter filling | 1 | 60 | 8 | Tr | 8 | 1 | 2 |
| vanilla w/ crème filling | 1 | 50 | 7 | Tr | 7 | Tr | 2 |
| Shortbread cookie, plain | 1 | 45 | 6 | Tr | 6 | Tr | 2 |
| w/ fudge stripes | 1 | 65 | 9 | Tr | 9 | Tr | 3 |
| Sugar Cookie, regular | 1 | 65 | 8 | Tr | 8 | 1 | 3 |
| reduced fat | 1 | 55 | 9 | Tr | 9 | 1 | 1 |
| Wafer, crème filled, 2 ½" x 1" rectangles, chocolate, | | | | | | | |
| crème filling | 3 | 140 | 18 | 1 | 17 | 1 | 7 |
| sugar-free, w/ filling | 3 | 100 | 14 | Tr | 14 | 1 | 8 |
| vanilla, crème filling | 3 | 130 | 19 | Tr | 19 | 1 | 6 |
| Wafer, Vanilla, round, 1 ½" dia | 4 | 75 | 10 | Tr | 10 | 1 | 3 |
| **Cooking Spray, nonstick** | | | | | | | |
| **¼ second spray** | **1 spray** | **0** | **0** | **0** | **0** | **0** | **0** |
| **Corn** | | | | | | | |
| Sweet White, 5" cob, cooked | 1 ear | 83 | 19 | 2 | 17 | 3 | 1 |
| Sweet Yellow, on 5" cob, fresh, cooked, 5" cob | 1 ear | 83 | 19 | 2 | 17 | 3 | 1 |

| | Serving Size | Calories (g) | Total Carbs(g) | Fiber (g) | Net Carbs(g) | Protein (g) | Fat (g) |
|---|---|---|---|---|---|---|---|
| frozen, cooked, 5" cob | 1 ear | 75 | 18 | 2 | 16 | 2 | 1 |
| frozen, cooked, kernels | ½ cup | 65 | 16 | 2 | 14 | 2 | Tr |
| canned, kernels, vacuum pack | ½ cup | 83 | 20 | 2 | 18 | 3 | 1 |
| canned, cream style kernels | ½ cup | 92 | 23 | 2 | 21 | 2 | 1 |
| Prep w/butter & herb sauce | ¾ cup | 180 | 30 | 2 | 28 | 5 | 4 |
| **Corn Cake,** butter flavor (also see Rice Cake) | 1 | 40 | 8 | 1 | 7 | 1 | Tr |
| **Corn Chips** | | | | | | | |
| Regular | 1 oz | 160 | 15 | 1 | 14 | 2 | 10 |
| Barbecue flavor | 1 oz | 170 | 17 | 1 | 16 | 2 | 10 |
| Ranch flavor | 1 oz | 150 | 20 | 1 | 19 | 2 | 7 |
| Reduced fat | 1 oz | 130 | 22 | 1 | 21 | 2 | 5 |
| Tortilla type | 1 oz | 140 | 17 | 1 | 16 | 2 | 7 |
| Doritos corn chips | 12 chips | 140 | 18 | 1 | 17 | 2 | 7 |
| nacho cheese | 12 chips | 140 | 18 | 1 | 17 | 2 | 7 |
| ranch | 12 chips | 140 | 18 | 1 | 17 | 2 | 7 |
| spicy nacho | 12 chips | 135 | 18 | 1 | 17 | 2 | 6 |
| Fritos corn chips, regular | 28 chips | 160 | 15 | 1 | 14 | 2 | 10 |
| BBQ corn chips | 28 chips | 160 | 16 | 1 | 15 | 2 | 9 |
| Chili cheese corn chips | 28 chips | 160 | 15 | 1 | 14 | 2 | 10 |
| Tostitos corn chips, round | 13 chips | 150 | 19 | 1 | 18 | 2 | 6 |
| baked | 13 chips | 110 | 21 | 1 | 20 | 3 | 1 |
| nacho | 6 chips | 150 | 19 | 1 | 18 | 2 | 6 |
| restaurant style | 7 chips | 140 | 19 | 1 | 18 | 2 | 6 |
| **Corn Grits (hominy)** – see Grits | ... | ... | . | . | . | . | . |
| **Corn Syrup** | 1 Tbsp | 56 | 15 | 0 | 15 | 0 | 0 |
| **Cornbread,** 3" x 2" | 1 piece | 185 | 29 | 1 | 28 | 4 | 6 |
| ***Corned Beef,* canned** | *3 oz* | *215* | *0* | *0* | *0* | *23* | *13* |
| **Corned Beef Hash** | 1 cup | 440 | 23 | 1 | 22 | 19 | 30 |
| ***Cornish Hen,* roasted** | *4 oz* | *200* | *0* | *0* | *0* | *19* | *14* |
| **Cornmeal,** yellow, dry form | | | | | | | |
| Whole grain | 1 cup | 440 | 94 | 9 | 85 | 10 | 4 |
| Self rising | 1 cup | 490 | 103 | 10 | 93 | 12 | 2 |

| | Serving Size | Calories (g) | Total Carbs(g) | Fiber (g) | Net Carbs(g) | Protein (g) | Fat (g) |
|---|---|---|---|---|---|---|---|
| **Cornstarch** | 1 Tbsp | 30 | 7 | Tr | 7 | Tr | Tr |
| **Cottage cheese –** see Cheese | ... | ... | . | . | . | . | . |
| **Crabcake** | 1 | 150 | 12 | Tr | 12 | 9 | 4 |
| **Cracker Jacks** | ½ cup | 120 | 23 | 2 | 21 | 2 | 2 |
| **CRACKERS** | | | | | | | |
| Butter flavor, round, 2" dia | 5 | 80 | 10 | Tr | 10 | 1 | 4 |
| Cheese crackers, 1" squares | 10 | 50 | 6 | Tr | 6 | 1 | 3 |
| Chicken in a Biskit | 12 | 160 | 17 | 1 | 16 | 2 | 8 |
| Club crackers | 4 | 70 | 9 | Tr | 9 | 1 | 3 |
| Keebler Club | 4 | 50 | 6 | Tr | 6 | Tr | 2 |
| Graham crackers, 2 ½" sq | 3 | 90 | 16 | Tr | 16 | 1 | 2 |
| Matzo, plain, 6" sq | 1 | 120 | 25 | 1 | 24 | 3 | Tr |
| Melba toast, plain | 4 | 80 | 15 | Tr | 15 | 2 | 1 |
| Oat Thins | 9 | 70 | 10 | 1 | 9 | 2 | 3 |
| Oyster crackers | 25 | 65 | 11 | 1 | 10 | 1 | 1 |
| Ritz Bitz w/peanut butter | 13 | 150 | 17 | 1 | 16 | 4 | 8 |
| Ritz crackers, regular | 5 | 80 | 10 | Tr | 10 | 1 | 4 |
| reduced fat | 5 | 70 | 11 | Tr | 11 | 1 | 2 |
| Saltine crackers | 4 | 50 | 9 | Tr | 9 | 1 | 1 |
| Sandwich crackers, 1 ½" dia, | | | | | | | |
| cheese filled | 2 | 65 | 8 | Tr | 8 | 2 | 2 |
| peanut butter filled | 2 | 68 | 8 | Tr | 8 | 2 | 4 |
| Snack crackers, round, 2" dia | 5 | 80 | 10 | Tr | 10 | 1 | 4 |
| *Sociables* | 7 | 80 | 9 | Tr | 9 | 1 | 4 |
| *Town House crackers* | 5 | 80 | 9 | Tr | 9 | 1 | 4 |
| *Triscuit wafers* | 7 | 140 | 21 | 1 | 20 | 3 | 5 |
| Vegetable crackers, thin squares | 7 | 80 | 10 | 1 | 9 | 2 | 4 |
| *Wheat Thins* | 9 | 60 | 10 | 1 | 9 | 1 | 2 |
| Wheatables | 8 | 70 | 10 | 1 | 9 | 1 | 3 |
| Whole wheat, thin squares | 8 | 75 | 10 | 1 | 9 | 2 | 4 |
| Zwieback | 2 | 70 | 12 | 1 | 11 | 2 | 2 |

| | Serving Size | Calories (g) | Total Carbs(g) | Fiber (g) | Net Carbs(g) | Protein (g) | Fat (g) |
|---|---|---|---|---|---|---|---|
| **Cranberries** | | | | | | | |
| ***Fresh, raw, unsweetened*** | ***½ cup*** | ***23*** | ***5*** | ***2*** | ***3*** | ***Tr*** | ***Tr*** |
| Dried, sweetened | ¼ cup | 90 | 24 | 3 | 21 | Tr | Tr |
| **Cranberry Relish** | ¾ cup | 330 | 70 | 2 | 68 | 1 | 5 |
| w/walnuts | ¾ cup | 365 | 75 | 3 | 72 | 3 | 6 |
| **Cranberry Sauce,** sweet, canned | 1 slice | 85 | 22 | 1 | 21 | Tr | Tr |
| **Cream Cheese** – see Cheese | ... | ... | . | . | . | . | . |
| ***Cream of Tartar*** | ***1 tsp*** | ***8*** | ***2*** | ***Tr*** | ***2*** | ***0*** | ***0*** |
| **Cream of Wheat** Cereal, as prep | 1 cup | 130 | 27 | 1 | 26 | 4 | Tr |
| **Cream, Whipped Topping** | | | | | | | |
| Light | 1 cup | 700 | 7 | 0 | 7 | 5 | 75 |
| ***Light*** | ***1 Tbsp*** | ***45*** | ***Tr*** | ***0*** | ***Tr*** | ***Tr*** | ***5*** |
| Heavy | 1 cup | 820 | 7 | 0 | 7 | 5 | 88 |
| ***Heavy*** | ***1 Tbsp*** | ***50*** | ***Tr*** | ***0*** | ***Tr*** | ***Tr*** | ***6*** |
| ***Pressurized in can*** | ***1 Tbsp*** | ***8*** | ***Tr*** | ***0*** | ***Tr*** | ***Tr*** | ***1*** |
| **Creamer** – see Beverages, Creamer | ... | ... | . | . | . | . | . |
| **Croissant**, butter flavor, 4" | 1 | 230 | 26 | 2 | 24 | 5 | 12 |
| **Croutons**, seasoned | ½ cup | 92 | 13 | 1 | 12 | 2 | 3 |
| **Cucumber** | | | | | | | |
| Fresh, peeled, whole, 8" long | 1 | 35 | 7 | 2 | 5 | 2 | Tr |
| ***Fresh, peeled, sliced*** | ***1 cup*** | ***14*** | ***3*** | ***1*** | ***2*** | ***1*** | ***Tr*** |
| Fresh, unpeeled, whole, 8" long | 1 | 40 | 8 | 2 | 6 | 2 | Tr |
| ***Fresh, unpeeled, sliced*** | ***1 cup*** | ***14*** | ***3*** | ***1*** | ***2*** | ***1*** | ***Tr*** |
| **Cucumber Salad,** mayo dressing | ¾ cup | 120 | 9 | 2 | 7 | 2 | 10 |
| **Cupcake**, w/frosting, avg size, 2 ¾" dia x 2 ¾" tall | | | | | | | |
| Banana | 1 | 190 | 32 | 1 | 31 | 1 | 6 |
| Blueberry | 1 | 185 | 30 | 1 | 29 | 1 | 6 |
| Chocolate | 1 | 195 | 32 | 1 | 31 | 2 | 6 |

| | Serving Size | Calories (g) | Total Carbs(g) | Fiber (g) | Net Carbs(g) | Protein (g) | Fat (g) |
|---|---|---|---|---|---|---|---|
| Chocolate w/ crème filling | 1 | 190 | 31 | 1 | 30 | 1 | 7 |
| Coconut w/ crème filling | 1 | 200 | 34 | 1 | 33 | 1 | 7 |
| Strawberry | 1 | 185 | 30 | 1 | 29 | 1 | 6 |
| Vanilla | 1 | 190 | 32 | Tr | 32 | 1 | 6 |
| *Curry Powder* | *1 tsp* | *7* | *1* | *Tr* | *Tr* | *Tr* | *Tr* |
| Custard | ½ cup | 170 | 23 | Tr | 23 | 6 | 6 |
| *Dandelion Greens, cooked* | *1 cup* | *35* | *7* | *3* | *4* | *2* | *Tr* |
| Danish Pastry | | | | | | | |
| Cheese, 4" dia | 1 | 265 | 26 | 1 | 25 | 6 | 15 |
| Cinnamon & raisin, 4" dia | 1 | 260 | 33 | 2 | 31 | 5 | 12 |
| Fruit filled, 4" dia | 1 | 260 | 34 | 1 | 33 | 4 | 12 |
| Large, Cheese w/ fruit, 5" x 3" | 1 | 425 | 55 | 2 | 53 | 8 | 18 |
| Dates, pitted | | | | | | | |
| Whole | 5 dates | 115 | 30 | 3 | 27 | 1 | Tr |
| Chopped | 1 cup | 490 | 130 | 13 | 117 | 4 | 1 |
| Dessert – see Ice Cream, Frozen Dessert, or specific listing | ... | ... | . | . | . | . | . |
| Dessert Filling – see specific listing | ... | ... | . | . | . | . | . |
| Dessert Topping – see Topping | ... | ... | . | . | . | . | . |
| *Dill Weed, raw, sprigs* | *5* | *Tr* | *Tr* | *Tr* | *Tr* | *Tr* | *Tr* |
| Dip | | | | | | | |
| *Avocado* | *1 Tbsp* | *30* | *2* | *Tr* | *2* | *1* | *2* |
| *Bacon* | *1 Tbsp* | *30* | *2* | *Tr* | *2* | *1* | *2* |
| *French Onion* | *1 Tbsp* | *25* | *1* | *Tr* | *1* | *Tr* | *2* |
| *Ranch* | *1 Tbsp* | *30* | *2* | *Tr* | *2* | *1* | *2* |
| *Sour Cream & Chives, regular* | *1 Tbsp* | *30* | *2* | *Tr* | *2* | *1* | *2* |
| *light* | *1 Tbsp* | *15* | *2* | *Tr* | *2* | *1* | *Tr* |
| Doughnut | | | | | | | |
| Cake Doughnuts | | | | | | | |
| Regular ring type, 3" dia | | | | | | | |
| Plain | 1 | 200 | 23 | 1 | 22 | 2 | 11 |

| | Serving Size | Calories (g) | Total Carbs(g) | Fiber (g) | Net Carbs(g) | Protein (g) | Fat (g) |
|---|---|---|---|---|---|---|---|
| Powdered sugar | 1 | 240 | 33 | 1 | 32 | 3 | 11 |
| Chocolate frosting | 1 | 270 | 36 | 1 | 35 | 3 | 13 |
| Vanilla frosting & sprinkles | 1 | 280 | 39 | 1 | 38 | 3 | 13 |
| *Holes or Munchkin type, small* | | | | | | | |
| Cinnamon coated | 4 | 250 | 30 | 2 | 28 | 3 | 14 |
| Plain | 4 | 220 | 22 | 2 | 20 | 2 | 14 |
| Powdered sugar | 4 | 250 | 29 | 2 | 27 | 2 | 14 |
| *Cruller* | | | | | | | |
| Glazed & frosted w/chocolate | 1 | 280 | 35 | 1 | 34 | 2 | 15 |
| **Yeast Doughnuts** | | | | | | | |
| *Regular ring type, 3" dia* | | | | | | | |
| Glazed | 1 | 200 | 22 | 1 | 21 | 2 | 12 |
| Glazed & frosted w/vanilla | 1 | 250 | 33 | 1 | 32 | 3 | 12 |
| Glazed & frosted w/chocolate plus sprinkles | 1 | 270 | 36 | 1 | 35 | 3 | 12 |
| *Holes or Munchkin type, small* | | | | | | | |
| Glazed | 5 | 200 | 27 | 1 | 26 | 3 | 9 |
| Sugar coated | 6 | 220 | 26 | 1 | 25 | 4 | 12 |
| *Filled doughnuts* | | | | | | | |
| Vanilla iced, crème filled | 1 | 360 | 41 | 2 | 39 | 5 | 19 |
| Powdered & strawberry filled | 1 | 260 | 26 | 1 | 25 | 3 | 16 |
| **Dressing** – see Salad Dressing | ... | ... | . | . | . | . | . |
| **Dried Fruit** – see specific listings, and Trail Mix | ... | ... | . | . | . | . | . |
| **Duck,** roasted | | | | | | | |
| *½ Duck, meat only* | *½ duck* | *445* | *0* | *0* | *0* | *52* | *25* |
| **Éclair,** 5" x 2" | 1 | 260 | 24 | 1 | 23 | 6 | 16 |
| **EGG** | | | | | | | |
| Raw Eggs | | | | | | | |
| *1 med whole egg* | *1* | *65* | *1* | *0* | *1* | *5* | *4* |
| *1 Lg whole egg* | *1* | *75* | *1* | *0* | *1* | *6* | *5* |

| | Serving Size | Calories (g) | Total Carbs(g) | Fiber (g) | Net Carbs(g) | Protein (g) | Fat (g) |
|---|---|---|---|---|---|---|---|
| **1 extra Lg** | | | | | | | |
| whole egg | 1 | 85 | 1 | 0 | 1 | 7 | 6 |
| 1 yolk only, Lg | 1 | 60 | Tr | 0 | Tr | 3 | 5 |
| 1 white only, Lg | 1 | 15 | Tr | 0 | Tr | 4 | 0 |
| Prepared Eggs | | | | | | | |
| (1 Lg egg/svg) | | | | | | | |
| deviled | 1 | 120 | 1 | 0 | 1 | 7 | 10 |
| hard boiled, whole | 1 | 75 | 1 | 0 | 1 | 6 | 5 |
| hard boiled, chopped | 1 cup | 210 | 2 | 0 | 2 | 17 | 14 |
| omelet, plain, | | | | | | | |
| milk added | 1 | 105 | 1 | 0 | 1 | 7 | 8 |
| pan fried in | | | | | | | |
| margarine | 1 | 92 | 1 | 0 | 1 | 6 | 7 |
| poached | 1 | 75 | 1 | 0 | 1 | 6 | 5 |
| scrambled | | | | | | | |
| w/margarine & milk | 1 | 100 | 1 | 0 | 1 | 7 | 7 |
| **Egg Substitute** | | | | | | | |
| **or imitation** | ¼ cup | 35 | Tr | 0 | Tr | 6 | 1 |
| Eggplant | | | | | | | |
| **Cubed, cooked** | 1 cup | 28 | 7 | 3 | 4 | 1 | Tr |
| Fried sticks | ½ cup | 240 | 28 | 3 | 25 | 4 | 12 |
| Eggplant Parmagiana | ½ cup | 265 | 26 | 3 | 23 | 6 | 16 |
| Eggroll | | | | | | | |
| Chicken, Chun King entrée | 1 meal | 170 | 25 | 2 | 23 | 7 | 5 |
| Chicken, La Choy entrée | 1 meal | 170 | 25 | 2 | 23 | 7 | 5 |
| Pork, Chun King entrée | 1 meal | 170 | 23 | 2 | 21 | 6 | 6 |
| Pork eggroll, 4" long, 1 avg | 1 | 165 | 22 | 2 | 20 | 6 | 6 |
| Shrimp, Chun King entrée | 1 meal | 150 | 24 | 2 | 22 | 6 | 4 |
| Enchilada | | | | | | | |
| Beef, Banquet entrée | 1 meal | 380 | 54 | 1 | 53 | 15 | 12 |
| Beef, Patio entrée | 1 meal | 350 | 52 | 1 | 51 | 12 | 10 |
| Cheese, Banquet entrée | 1 meal | 340 | 56 | 1 | 55 | 15 | 6 |
| Chicken, Banquet entrée | 1 meal | 360 | 54 | 1 | 53 | 15 | 10 |
| Enchirito | | | | | | | |
| Beef | 1 | 370 | 33 | 2 | 31 | 18 | 19 |
| Chicken | 1 | 350 | 32 | 2 | 30 | 21 | 16 |
| Steak | 1 | 350 | 31 | 2 | 29 | 22 | 16 |
| **Endive, raw, chopped** | 1 cup | 9 | 2 | 2 | 0 | 1 | Tr |
| Energy Bar, low carb | | | | | | | |

| | Serving Size | Calories (g) | Total Carbs(g) | Fiber (g) | Net Carbs(g) | Protein (g) | Fat (g) |
|---|---|---|---|---|---|---|---|
| *Atkins Advantage* | | | | | | | |
| **Chocolate** | *1 bar* | *220* | *25* | *11* | *3* | *17* | *11* |
| *Atkins Advantage* | | | | | | | |
| **S'mores** | *1 bar* | *220* | *26* | *11* | *3* | *17* | *10* |
| *(net carbs as per manufacturer)* | | | | | | | |
| **English Muffin**, regular | 1 whole | 135 | 26 | 2 | 24 | 4 | 1 |
| Cinnamon raisin | 1 whole | 140 | 28 | 2 | 26 | 4 | 2 |
| *Equal sweetener* | *1 pkt* | *0* | *Tr* | *0* | *Tr* | *0* | *0* |
| **Fajita,** | | | | | | | |
| Chicken, *Healthy Choice* | 1 meal | 260 | 36 | 1 | 35 | 21 | 4 |
| **Fettuccini Alfredo,** w/ beef | 1 cup | 310 | 26 | 2 | 24 | 20 | 13 |
| **Fig,** fresh or dried, Lg | 2 | 98 | 25 | 5 | 20 | 1 | Tr |
| **FISH / SEAFOOD** | | | | | | | |
| Abalone, fried | 3 oz | 160 | 9 | 1 | 8 | 17 | 6 |
| *Anchovy, canned in oil* | *5* | *42* | *0* | *0* | *0* | *6* | *2* |
| Bass | | | | | | | |
| black, baked | 3 oz | 260 | 11 | 0 | 11 | 16 | 16 |
| **striped, baked** | *3 oz* | *105* | *0* | *0* | *0* | *19* | *3* |
| *Bluefish, baked* | *3 oz* | *135* | *0* | *0* | *0* | *22* | *5* |
| Catfish | | | | | | | |
| **baked or broiled** | *3 oz* | *130* | *0* | *0* | *0* | *20* | *5* |
| breaded, fried | 3 oz | 195 | 17 | 1 | 16 | 13 | 8 |
| *Caviar, black or red* | *2 Tbsp* | *80* | *1* | *0* | *1* | *8* | *6* |
| Clams | | | | | | | |
| breaded, fried | ¾ cup | 450 | 39 | Tr | 39 | 13 | 26 |
| **canned, drained** | *3 oz* | *125* | *4* | *0* | *4* | *22* | *2* |
| canned, drained | 1 cup | 235 | 8 | 0 | 8 | 41 | 3 |
| *raw* | *3 oz* | *63* | *2* | *0* | *2* | *11* | *1* |
| *raw* | *1 med* | *11* | *Tr* | *0* | *Tr* | *2* | *Tr* |
| *steamed* | *3 oz* | *125* | *4* | *0* | *4* | *22* | *2* |
| *Cod, baked or broiled* | *3 oz* | *90* | *0* | *0* | *0* | *20* | *1* |
| Crab, | | | | | | | |
| Alaska king | | | | | | | |
| **steamed** | *3 oz* | *82* | *0* | *0* | *0* | *16* | *1* |
| **steamed** | *1 leg* | *130* | *0* | *0* | *0* | *26* | *2* |
| Blue | | | | | | | |
| **steamed** | *3 oz* | *88* | *0* | *0* | *0* | *17* | *2* |
| **canned** | *1 cup* | *135* | *0* | *0* | *0* | *28* | *2* |

| | Serving Size | Calories (g) | Total Carbs(g) | Fiber (g) | Net Carbs(g) | Protein (g) | Fat (g) |
|---|---|---|---|---|---|---|---|
| Crab meat, Imitation | 3 oz | 88 | 9 | 0 | 9 | 10 | 1 |
| *Crab cake, w/egg, fried* | *1 cake* | *95* | *1* | *0* | *1* | *12* | *5* |
| Fish fillet, breaded, fried | 3 oz | 190 | 17 | 1 | 16 | 10 | 9 |
| Fish stick, breaded, fried, 3" x 1" | 2 sticks | 76 | 7 | Tr | 7 | 4 | 3 |
| Flounder | | | | | | | |
| *baked or broiled* | *3 oz* | *100* | *0* | *0* | *0* | *21* | *1* |
| breaded, fried fillet | 3 oz | 190 | 17 | 1 | 16 | 13 | 8 |
| Grouper | | | | | | | |
| *baked or broiled* | *3 oz* | *100* | *0* | *0* | *0* | *21* | *1* |
| Haddock | | | | | | | |
| *baked or broiled* | *3 oz* | *95* | *0* | *0* | *0* | *21* | *1* |
| breaded, fried fillet | 3 oz | 195 | 17 | 1 | 16 | 13 | 8 |
| Halibut | | | | | | | |
| *baked or broiled* | *3 oz* | *120* | *0* | *0* | *0* | *23* | *2* |
| breaded, fried fillet | 3 oz | 210 | 17 | 1 | 16 | 14 | 9 |
| Herring, pickled | 3 oz | 225 | 8 | 0 | 8 | 12 | 15 |
| Lobster | | | | | | | |
| *steamed* | *3 oz* | *85* | *1* | *0* | *1* | *17* | *1* |
| imitation meat | 3 oz | 90 | 9 | 0 | 9 | 10 | 1 |
| Mackerel | ... | ... | . | . | . | . | . |
| *baked or broiled* | *3 oz* | *225* | *0* | *0* | *0* | *20* | *15* |
| *jack, canned* | *1 cup* | *295* | *0* | *0* | *0* | *44* | *12* |
| Monkfish, | | | | | | | |
| *baked or broiled* | *3 oz* | *130* | *0* | *0* | *0* | *21* | *4* |
| Mussels, steamed | 3 oz | 145 | 6 | 0 | 6 | 20 | 4 |
| *Orange roughy, baked or broiled* | *3 oz* | *75* | *0* | *0* | *0* | *16* | *1* |
| Oyster | | | | | | | |
| raw meat | 1 cup | 170 | 10 | 0 | 10 | 17 | 6 |
| *raw meat* | *6 med* | *55* | *3* | *0* | *3* | *6* | *2* |
| breaded, fried | 3 oz | 165 | 10 | 1 | 9 | 7 | 11 |
| *Perch, baked or broiled* | *3 oz* | *105* | *0* | *0* | *0* | *20* | *2* |
| *Pike, baked or broiled* | *3 oz* | *95* | *0* | *0* | *0* | *21* | *1* |
| *Pollock, baked or broiled* | *3 oz* | *95* | *0* | *0* | *0* | *20* | *1* |
| Pompano | | | | | | | |
| *baked or broiled* | *3 oz* | *180* | *0* | *0* | *0* | *20* | *10* |
| Rockfish | | | | | | | |
| *baked or broiled* | *3 oz* | *105* | *0* | *0* | *0* | *20* | *2* |

| | Serving Size | Calories (g) | Total Carbs(g) | Fiber (g) | Net Carbs(g) | Protein (g) | Fat (g) |
|---|---|---|---|---|---|---|---|
| Salmon | | | | | | | |
| **baked or broiled** | **3 oz** | **185** | **0** | **0** | **0** | **23** | **9** |
| **canned, pink** | **3 oz** | **118** | **0** | **0** | **0** | **17** | **5** |
| **smoked, chinook** | **3 oz** | **100** | **0** | **0** | **0** | **16** | **4** |
| **Sardine, canned in oil,** | | | | | | | |
| **drained** | **3 oz** | **175** | **0** | **0** | **0** | **21** | **10** |
| Scallop | | | | | | | |
| breaded, fried | 6 large | 200 | 9 | Tr | 9 | 17 | 10 |
| **steamed** | **3 oz** | **95** | **3** | **0** | **3** | **20** | **1** |
| Shark | | | | | | | |
| **Pacific shark, baked** | **3 oz** | **130** | **0** | **0** | **0** | **15** | **8** |
| **thrasher, baked** | **3 oz** | **85** | **0** | **0** | **0** | **18** | **1** |
| Shrimp | | | | | | | |
| breaded, fried | 2 large | 110 | 5 | Tr | 5 | 10 | 6 |
| breaded, fried | 3 oz | 205 | 10 | Tr | 10 | 18 | 10 |
| **canned, drained** | **3 oz** | **100** | **1** | **0** | **1** | **20** | **2** |
| **steamed** | **3 oz** | **84** | **0** | **0** | **0** | **18** | **1** |
| **Snapper, baked** | | | | | | | |
| **or broiled** | **3 oz** | **110** | **0** | **0** | **0** | **22** | **2** |
| Sole | | | | | | | |
| **baked or broiled** | **3 oz** | **100** | **0** | **0** | **0** | **21** | **1** |
| breaded, fried fillet | 3 oz | 190 | 17 | 1 | 16 | 13 | 8 |
| Squid, fried | 3 oz | 150 | 7 | 0 | 7 | 15 | 6 |
| Swordfish | | | | | | | |
| **baked** | **3 oz** | **130** | **0** | **0** | **0** | **22** | **4** |
| **broiled** | **4 oz** | **170** | **0** | **0** | **0** | **28** | **5** |
| **Trout, baked or broiled** | **3 oz** | **145** | **0** | **0** | **0** | **21** | **6** |
| Tuna | | | | | | | |
| **baked or broiled** | **3 oz** | **120** | **0** | **0** | **0** | **25** | **1** |
| **canned in oil, drained** | **3 oz** | **170** | **0** | **0** | **0** | **25** | **7** |
| **canned in water,** | | | | | | | |
| **chunk light** | **3 oz** | **100** | **0** | **0** | **0** | **22** | **1** |
| **canned in water,** | | | | | | | |
| **solid white** | **3 oz** | **110** | **0** | **0** | **0** | **20** | **3** |
| tuna salad, oil packed, w/mayo | ½ cup | 190 | 9 | 0 | 9 | 16 | 10 |
| tuna salad, water packed, w/light mayo | | | | | | | |
| type dressing | ½ cup | 130 | 6 | 0 | 6 | 15 | 5 |
| **Whiting, baked** | | | | | | | |
| **or broiled** | **3 oz** | **100** | **0** | **0** | **0** | **21** | **1** |

| | Serving Size | Calories (g) | Total Carbs(g) | Fiber (g) | Net Carbs(g) | Protein (g) | Fat (g) |
|---|---|---|---|---|---|---|---|
| **Fish & Chips,** *Swanson entrée* | 1 meal | 495 | 60 | 2 | 58 | 20 | 20 |
| **Fish & Macaroni w/cheese** *Stouffers entrée* | 1 meal | 460 | 47 | 2 | 45 | 22 | 20 |
| **Fish Baked w/Lemon Pepper** *Healthy Choice entrée* | 1 meal | 290 | 47 | 1 | 46 | 14 | 5 |
| **Fish Florentine,** *Lean Cuisine* | 1 meal | 240 | 13 | Tr | 13 | 27 | 9 |
| **Fish Sandwich,** 3 oz fried fish fillet w/ tarter sauce & cheese | 1 avg | 530 | 48 | Tr | 48 | 22 | 29 |
| **Flank Steak** – see Beef | ... | ... | . | . | . | . | . |
| **Flour,** unsifted | | | | | | | |
| All purpose flour, white | 1 cup | 455 | 95 | 3 | 92 | 13 | 1 |
| Bread flour | 1 cup | 495 | 99 | 3 | 96 | 16 | 2 |
| Buckwheat flour, whole groat | 1 cup | 400 | 85 | 12 | 73 | 15 | 4 |
| Cake or pastry flour | 1 cup | 495 | 107 | 2 | 105 | 11 | 1 |
| Carob flour | 1 cup | 230 | 92 | 41 | 51 | 5 | 1 |
| Self-rising flour, white | 1 cup | 443 | 93 | 3 | 90 | 12 | 1 |
| Whole wheat flour | 1 cup | 407 | 87 | 15 | 72 | 16 | 2 |
| **Frankfurter** – see Hot Dog | ... | ... | . | . | . | . | . |
| **Freezer Pop** – see Frozen Dessert | ... | ... | . | . | . | . | . |
| **French Fries** *Frozen, heated,* thin, shoestring strips, 3 oz | 20 fries | 130 | 22 | 2 | 20 | 2 | 4 |
| thick or crinkle cuts, 4.5 oz | 20 fries | 195 | 33 | 3 | 30 | 3 | 6 |
| Restaurant type, regular fries | 1 med | 350 | 48 | 5 | 43 | 5 | 15 |
| Curly Cheddar Fries | 1 med | 460 | 54 | 5 | 49 | 6 | 24 |
| Curly Fries | 1 med | 400 | 40 | 5 | 35 | 5 | 20 |
| **French Toast** | 2 slices | 250 | 38 | 1 | 37 | 8 | 8 |
| **Fried Chicken** – see Chicken | ... | ... | . | . | . | . | . |

| | Serving Size | Calories (g) | Total Carbs(g) | Fiber (g) | Net Carbs(g) | Protein (g) | Fat (g) |
|---|---|---|---|---|---|---|---|
| **Fried Rice** – see Rice | ... | ... | . | . | . | . | . |
| **Frijoles** | 1 cup | 225 | 29 | 2 | 27 | 11 | 8 |
| **Frosting** | | | | | | | |
| Chocolate | 1 Tbsp | 75 | 12 | Tr | 12 | Tr | 3 |
| Vanilla | 1 Tbsp | 80 | 13 | Tr | 13 | Tr | 3 |
| **Frozen Dessert** | | | | | | | |
| (also see Ice Cream) | | | | | | | |
| Freezer Pop – (long tubes) | | | | | | | |
| Regular, fruit flavored, 1.5 oz | 1 | 25 | 6 | 0 | 6 | 0 | 0 |
| *Sugar-free, fruit flavored, 1.5 oz* | *2* | *4* | *1* | *0* | *1* | *0* | *0* |
| Frozen chocolate log cake | 1 slice | 280 | 43 | 1 | 42 | 5 | 9 |
| Frozen chocolate round cake | 1 slice | 340 | 53 | 1 | 52 | 7 | 12 |
| Fruit & Juice bar, 2.5 oz | 1 | 65 | 16 | 0 | 16 | 1 | Tr |
| Fudge bar, 1.75 oz | 1 | 65 | 13 | Tr | 13 | 4 | Tr |
| Ice pop bar, 2 oz | 1 | 45 | 11 | 0 | 11 | 0 | 0 |
| Italian ices | ½ cup | 65 | 16 | 0 | 16 | Tr | Tr |
| Popsicle, 4 oz | 1 | 90 | 22 | 0 | 22 | 0 | 0 |
| Vanilla sandwich bar | 1 | 220 | 31 | 1 | 30 | 4 | 9 |
| **Fruit** (see specific listings) | | | | | | | |
| Mixed, canned, w/light syrup | 1 cup | 150 | 39 | 2 | 37 | 2 | Tr |
| Mixed, frozen, sweetened | 1 cup | 245 | 61 | 5 | 56 | 4 | Tr |
| **Fruit Cocktail** | | | | | | | |
| Canned in heavy syrup | 1 cup | 180 | 47 | 3 | 42 | 1 | Tr |
| Canned in juice | 1 cup | 110 | 28 | 2 | 26 | 1 | Tr |
| **Fruit Salad,** mixed diced fruits | ¾ cup | 70 | 9 | 3 | 6 | 1 | 1 |
| **Fudge** | | | | | | | |
| Chocolate fudge, plain | 1 oz | 110 | 24 | Tr | 24 | 1 | 2 |
| Chocolate fudge w/ nuts | 1 oz | 125 | 21 | Tr | 21 | 2 | 4 |
| Vanilla fudge, plain | 1 oz | 105 | 23 | Tr | 23 | 1 | 1 |
| Vanilla fudge, w/nuts | 1 oz | 120 | 22 | Tr | 22 | 1 | 4 |
| *Funyuns* (snacks) | 13 | 140 | 18 | 1 | 17 | 2 | 7 |
| *Garlic, raw* | *1 clove* | *4* | *1* | *Tr* | *Tr* | *Tr* | *Tr* |
| *Garlic Powder or Salt* | *1 tsp* | *8* | *2* | *Tr* | *2* | *Tr* | *Tr* |

| | Serving Size | Calories (g) | Total Carbs (g) | Fiber (g) | Net Carbs (g) | Protein (g) | Fat (g) |
|---|---|---|---|---|---|---|---|
| **Gelatin** *(Jello)* | | | | | | | |
| Banana, regular | ½ cup | 80 | 19 | 0 | 19 | 2 | 0 |
| ***Banana, sugar free*** | *½ cup* | *10* | *1* | *0* | *1* | *1* | *0* |
| Cherry, regular | ½ cup | 75 | 18 | 0 | 18 | 2 | 0 |
| ***Cherry, sugar free*** | *½ cup* | *10* | *1* | *0* | *1* | *1* | *0* |
| Orange, regular | ½ cup | 75 | 18 | 0 | 18 | 2 | 0 |
| ***Orange, sugar free*** | *½ cup* | *10* | *1* | *0* | *1* | *1* | *0* |
| Raspberry, regular | ½ cup | 75 | 18 | 0 | 18 | 2 | 0 |
| ***Raspberry, sugar free*** | *½ cup* | *10* | *1* | *0* | *1* | *1* | *0* |
| Strawberry , regular | ½ cup | 75 | 18 | 0 | 18 | 2 | 0 |
| ***Strawberry, sugar free*** | *½ cup* | *10* | *1* | *0* | *1* | *1* | *0* |
| **Gordita** | | | | | | | |
| Beef & cheese | 1 | 310 | 30 | 2 | 28 | 13 | 15 |
| Chicken & cheese | 1 | 290 | 29 | 2 | 27 | 15 | 13 |
| Steak & cheese | 1 | 290 | 28 | 2 | 26 | 16 | 13 |
| **Granola Bar** | | | | | | | |
| Low fat, fruit variety | 1 bar | 90 | 19 | 2 | 17 | 3 | 1 |
| Plain granola bar | 1 bar | 135 | 18 | 2 | 16 | 3 | 6 |
| Chocolate chip | 1 bar | 150 | 22 | 1 | 21 | 3 | 6 |
| Chocolate chip & peanuts | 1 bar | 160 | 18 | 2 | 16 | 4 | 10 |
| Coconut | 1 bar | 140 | 20 | 1 | 19 | 3 | 6 |
| Raisin | 1 bar | 140 | 20 | 1 | 19 | 3 | 6 |
| **Grapefruit,** pink, red, or white | | | | | | | |
| fresh, 3 ¾" dia | 1 | 80 | 18 | 3 | 15 | 2 | Tr |
| canned, in juice | 1 cup | 115 | 28 | 2 | 26 | 1 | Tr |
| canned, in light syrup | 1 cup | 150 | 39 | 1 | 38 | 1 | Tr |
| **Grapes,** seeded Fresh, medium size, | | | | | | | |
| all types | 10 grapes | 35 | 9 | 1 | 8 | Tr | Tr |
| Fresh, small or medium size | 1 cup | 115 | 28 | 2 | 26 | 1 | 1 |
| **Gravy** | | | | | | | |
| ***Beef*** | *¼ cup* | *40* | *4* | *Tr* | *4* | *2* | *2* |
| ***Chicken*** | *¼ cup* | *32* | *3* | *Tr* | *3* | *2* | *1* |
| ***Country Sausage*** | *¼ cup* | *60* | *4* | *Tr* | *4* | *2* | *4* |
| ***Mushroom*** | *¼ cup* | *30* | *3* | *Tr* | *3* | *1* | *2* |
| ***Pork*** | *¼ cup* | *38* | *3* | *Tr* | *3* | *2* | *2* |
| ***Turkey*** | *¼ cup* | *31* | *3* | *Tr* | *3* | *2* | *1* |

| | Serving Size | Calories (g) | Total Carbs(g) | Fiber (g) | Net Carbs(g) | Protein (g) | Fat (g) |
|---|---|---|---|---|---|---|---|
| **Grits,** corn (hominy), as prep | 1 cup | 145 | 31 | 1 | 30 | 3 | Tr |
| **Ground Beef** – see Beef | ... | ... | . | . | . | . | . |
| **Guava,** raw, med size | 1 | 45 | 11 | 2 | 9 | 1 | Tr |
| **Gum** – see Chewing Gum | ... | ... | . | . | . | . | . |
| **HAM** (also see Pork) | | | | | | | |
| *Canned, regular,* | | | | | | | |
| *roasted* | *3 oz* | *155* | *2* | *0* | *2* | *15* | *9* |
| *lean, roasted* | *3 oz* | *130* | *1* | *0* | *1* | *16* | *7* |
| *Leg, roasted, lean & fat* | *3 oz* | *230* | *0* | *0* | *0* | *23* | *15* |
| *lean only* | *3 oz* | *180* | *0* | *0* | *0* | *25* | *8* |
| *Light cure,* | | | | | | | |
| *roasted, lean & fat* | *3 oz* | *205* | *0* | *0* | *0* | *18* | *14* |
| *lean only* | *3 oz* | *135* | *0* | *0* | *0* | *21* | *5* |
| Lunch meat, 1/8" slices | | | | | | | |
| *regular* | *2 slices* | *150* | *3* | *0* | *3* | *21* | *5* |
| *lean/ lowfat* | *2 slices* | *60* | *2* | *0* | *2* | *10* | *1* |
| *baked* | *2 slices* | *100* | *2* | *0* | *2* | *16* | *2* |
| maple glazed | 2 slices | 120 | 6 | Tr | 6 | 18 | 2 |
| *smoked* | *2 slices* | *110* | *4* | *0* | *4* | *18* | *2* |
| **Hamburger & Cheeseburger** | | | | | | | |
| *w/ catsup, mustard, lettuce, & onion or pickle* | | | | | | | |
| 4 oz burger w/o cheese | 1 | 420 | 37 | 2 | 35 | 23 | 20 |
| 4 oz burger w/cheese | 1 | 530 | 38 | 2 | 36 | 28 | 30 |
| 2 oz burger w/o cheese | 1 | 260 | 32 | 2 | 30 | 14 | 9 |
| 2 oz burger w/cheese | 1 | 340 | 35 | 2 | 33 | 16 | 15 |
| (also, see Beef- Ground & Fast Food Restaurants) | ... | ... | . | . | . | . | . |
| **Hamburger Helper** | | | | | | | |
| Beef Pasta | 1 cup | 270 | 26 | 2 | 24 | 20 | 10 |
| Beef Romanoff | 1 cup | 290 | 28 | 2 | 26 | 20 | 11 |
| Beef Taco | 1 cup | 310 | 31 | 2 | 29 | 21 | 13 |
| Beef Teriyaki | 1 cup | 290 | 34 | 2 | 32 | 18 | 10 |
| Cheesy Shells | 1 cup | 340 | 30 | 2 | 28 | 22 | 14 |
| Fettuccini Alfredo | 1 cup | 310 | 26 | 2 | 24 | 20 | 13 |
| Zesty Italian | 1 cup | 320 | 34 | 2 | 32 | 21 | 11 |

| | Serving Size | Calories (g) | Total Carbs(g) | Fiber (g) | Net Carbs(g) | Protein (g) | Fat (g) |
|---|---|---|---|---|---|---|---|
| **Hash Browns** – see Potatoes | ... | ... | . | . | . | . | . |
| ***Hearts of Palm, canned*** | ***1 piece*** | ***9*** | ***2*** | ***1*** | ***1*** | ***1*** | ***Tr*** |
| Honey | 1 Tbsp | 64 | 17 | Tr | 17 | Tr | 0 |
| | 1 cup | 1030 | 279 | 1 | 278 | 1 | 0 |
| **Honeydew Melon** Fresh, avg size 6 ½" melon, | | | | | | | |
| cubed or diced | 1 cup | 60 | 16 | 1 | 15 | 1 | Tr |
| wedge, 1/8 of melon | 1 wedge | 55 | 15 | 1 | 14 | 1 | Tr |
| ***Horseradish, as prep*** | ***1 tsp*** | ***4*** | ***1*** | ***Tr*** | ***Tr*** | ***Tr*** | ***Tr*** |
| HOT DOG (FRANKFURTER) | | | | | | | |
| ***Beef or Pork*** | ***1*** | ***145*** | ***1*** | ***0*** | ***1*** | ***5*** | ***13*** |
| ***Chicken or Turkey*** | ***1*** | ***115*** | ***2*** | ***0*** | ***2*** | ***6*** | ***10*** |
| ***Lowfat, any meat*** | ***1*** | ***75*** | ***3*** | ***0*** | ***3*** | ***5*** | ***5*** |
| Fat free, any meat | 1 | 45 | 5 | 0 | 5 | 6 | 0 |
| **Hot Dog** (meal as prep) Hot Dog on Bun | | | | | | | |
| w/ catsup & mustard | 1 avg | 245 | 19 | 1 | 18 | 10 | 15 |
| Hot Dog on Bun w/ chili | 1 avg | 295 | 31 | 1 | 30 | 14 | 13 |
| Corndog | 1 avg | 395 | 49 | 2 | 47 | 16 | 16 |
| ***Hummus, commercial*** | ***1 Tbsp*** | ***23*** | ***2*** | ***1*** | ***1*** | ***1*** | ***1*** |
| **Hush Puppies** | 5 | 260 | 35 | 2 | 33 | 5 | 12 |
| **Ice Cream** Chocolate | | | | | | | |
| regular | ½ cup | 145 | 19 | 1 | 18 | 3 | 7 |
| reduced fat | ½ cup | 100 | 15 | 1 | 14 | 3 | 3 |
| Vanilla | | | | | | | |
| regular | ½ cup | 135 | 16 | 0 | 16 | 2 | 7 |
| reduced fat | ½ cup | 90 | 15 | 0 | 15 | 3 | 3 |
| rich | ½ cup | 180 | 17 | 0 | 17 | 3 | 12 |
| soft ice cream in cone | 1 cone | 200 | 19 | 0 | 19 | 4 | 13 |
| soft ice cream in cone, chocolate dipped | 1 cone | 255 | 32 | 1 | 31 | 5 | 13 |
| Sherbet, Orange | ½ cup | 100 | 22 | 0 | 22 | 1 | 1 |
| ***Ice Cream Cone, 2 ½" cup only*** | ***1 cup*** | ***20*** | ***4*** | ***0*** | ***4*** | ***0*** | ***0*** |
| **Ice Cream Sandwich,** vanilla | 1 | 220 | 31 | 1 | 30 | 4 | 9 |

| | Serving Size | Calories (g) | Total Carbs(g) | Fiber (g) | Net Carbs(g) | Protein (g) | Fat (g) |
|---|---|---|---|---|---|---|---|
| **Ice Pop** | ... | ... | . | . | . | . | . |
| – See Frozen Dessert | | | | | | | |
| Italian Ices | ½ cup | 65 | 16 | 0 | 16 | Tr | Tr |
| *Italian Seasoning,* *dried spice* | *1/2 tsp* | *3* | *Tr* | *Tr* | *Tr* | *Tr* | *0* |
| Jalapeno – see Peppers | ... | ... | . | . | . | . | . |
| Jam | | | | | | | |
| All flavors, regular | 1 Tbsp | 55 | 14 | Tr | 14 | Tr | Tr |
| All flavors, restaurant packet | 1 pkt | 39 | 10 | Tr | 10 | Tr | Tr |
| *Jello* – see Gelatin | ... | ... | . | . | . | . | . |
| Jelly | | | | | | | |
| All flavors, regular | 1 Tbsp | 54 | 13 | Tr | 13 | Tr | Tr |
| All flavors, restaurant packet | 1 pkt | 40 | 10 | Tr | 10 | Tr | Tr |
| Kale | | | | | | | |
| *Fresh, raw* | *1 cup* | *17* | *4* | *2* | *2* | *1* | *Tr* |
| *Fresh, chopped, cooked* | *1 cup* | *36* | *7* | *3* | *4* | *2* | *Tr* |
| *Frozen, chopped, cooked* | *1 cup* | *39* | *7* | *3* | *4* | *3* | *Tr* |
| *Ketchup, regular* | *1 Tbsp* | *18* | *4* | *Tr* | *4* | *Tr* | *Tr* |
| *restaurant size packet* | *1 pkt* | *10* | *3* | *Tr* | *3* | *Tr* | *Tr* |
| Kiwi fruit, fresh, medium size | 1 | 45 | 11 | 3 | 8 | 1 | Tr |
| *Knockwurst, beef,* *Boars Head* | *1 wurst* | *310* | *1* | *Tr* | *Tr* | *15* | *27* |
| Kohlrabi, cooked, slices | 1 cup | 48 | 11 | 2 | 9 | 3 | Tr |
| Lamb *(Braised, broiled, or roasted)* | | | | | | | |
| *Arm chop, lean & fat* | *3 oz* | *295* | *0* | *0* | *0* | *26* | *20* |
| *lean only* | *3 oz* | *235* | *0* | *0* | *0* | *30* | *12* |
| *Leg of lamb, lean & fat* | *3 oz* | *220* | *0* | *0* | *0* | *22* | *14* |
| *lean only* | *3 oz* | *160* | *0* | *0* | *0* | *24* | *7* |
| *Loin chop, lean & fat* | *3 oz* | *270* | *0* | *0* | *0* | *21* | *20* |
| *lean only* | *3 oz* | *185* | *0* | *0* | *0* | *25* | *8* |
| *Rib roast, lean & fat* | *3 oz* | *305* | *0* | *0* | *0* | *18* | *25* |
| *lean only* | *3 oz* | *195* | *0* | *0* | *0* | *22* | *11* |

| | Serving Size | Calories (g) | Total Carbs(g) | Fiber (g) | Net Carbs(g) | Protein (g) | Fat (g) |
|---|---|---|---|---|---|---|---|
| *Lard* | *1 cup* | *1850* | *0* | *0* | *0* | *0* | *205* |
| | *1 Tbsp* | *115* | *0* | *0* | *0* | *0* | *13* |
| **Lasagna**, avg size 2½" x 4" | | | | | | | |
| w/ meat sauce | 1 | 360 | 52 | 2 | 50 | 18 | 12 |
| w/ zucchini | 1 | 330 | 58 | 3 | 55 | 20 | 2 |
| **Leek**, chopped, cooked | 1 cup | 32 | 8 | 1 | 7 | 1 | Tr |
| *Lemon, fresh, 2 1/4" dia* | *1* | *20* | *4* | *2* | *2* | *1* | *Tr* |
| **Lentil**, cooked | ½ cup | 115 | 20 | 8 | 12 | 9 | 1 |
| **Lettuce**, fresh, raw | | | | | | | |
| Bibb, Boston, Butterhead | | | | | | | |
| **whole head, 5" dia** | **1 head** | **21** | **4** | **2** | **2** | **2** | **Tr** |
| **single leaf** | **1 leaf** | **1** | **Tr** | **Tr** | **Tr** | **Tr** | **Tr** |
| Iceberg, Crisphead | | | | | | | |
| **whole head, 6" dia** | **1 head** | **65** | **11** | **8** | **3** | **5** | **1** |
| **single leaf** | **1 leaf** | **1** | **Tr** | **Tr** | **Tr** | **Tr** | **Tr** |
| **pieces, chopped or shredded** | **1 cup** | **8** | **1** | **Tr** | **Tr** | **1** | **Tr** |
| **wedge slice, 1/6 of 6" head** | **1 wedge** | **11** | **2** | **1** | **1** | **1** | **Tr** |
| Loose leaf | | | | | | | |
| **single leaf** | **1 leaf** | **2** | **Tr** | **Tr** | **Tr** | **Tr** | **Tr** |
| **pieces, shredded or chopped** | **1 cup** | **10** | **2** | **1** | **1** | **1** | **Tr** |
| Romaine or cos | | | | | | | |
| **innerleaf** | **1 leaf** | **1** | **Tr** | **Tr** | **Tr** | **Tr** | **Tr** |
| **pieces, shredded** | **1 cup** | **8** | **1** | **Tr** | **Tr** | **1** | **Tr** |
| *Lime, fresh, 2" dia* | *1* | *20* | *5* | *2* | *3* | *Tr* | *Tr* |
| **Linguini w/Clam sauce** | | | | | | | |
| *Lean Cuisine entrée* | 1 meal | 260 | 32 | 2 | 30 | 16 | 7 |
| **Liver** | | | | | | | |
| Beef liver, fried | 3 oz | 185 | 7 | 0 | 7 | 23 | 7 |
| *Chicken liver, simmered* | *1 liver* | *31* | *Tr* | *0* | *Tr* | *5* | *1* |
| *Veal liver, braised* | *3.5 oz* | *165* | *0* | *0* | *0* | *22* | *7* |
| *Liverwurst, Boars Head* | *2 oz* | *170* | *1* | *Tr* | *Tr* | *8* | *15* |
| **Lobster** – see Fish / Seafood | ... | ... | . | . | . | . | . |
| **Lo Mein w/Vegetables** | 1½ cups | 230 | 40 | 3 | 37 | 8 | 4 |

| | Serving Size | Calories (g) | Total Carbs(g) | Fiber (g) | Net Carbs(g) | Protein (g) | Fat (g) |
|---|---|---|---|---|---|---|---|
| Lo Mein w/meat & vegetables | 1½ cups | 310 | 35 | 1 | 34 | 13 | 12 |
| Lunch Meat *(⅛" slices)* | | | | | | | |
| **Beef or Pork, regular** | **2 slices** | **180** | **2** | **0** | **2** | **7** | **16** |
| **Beef or Pork, lowfat** | **2 slices** | **110** | **2** | **0** | **2** | **6** | **9** |
| **Beef or Pork, fat free** | **2 slices** | **60** | **3** | **0** | **3** | **8** | **1** |
| **Chicken or Turkey, regular** | **2 slices** | **160** | **2** | **0** | **2** | **7** | **14** |
| **Chicken or Turkey, lowfat** | **2 slices** | **100** | **2** | **0** | **2** | **6** | **8** |
| **Chicken or Turkey, fat free** | **2 slices** | **60** | **3** | **0** | **3** | **8** | **1** |
| **Ham, regular** | **2 slices** | **150** | **3** | **0** | **3** | **21** | **5** |
| **Ham, lean/lowfat** | **2 slices** | **60** | **2** | **0** | **2** | **10** | **1** |
| (also see specific listings) | | | | | | | |
| Macaroni, elbows | | | | | | | |
| Dry, uncooked | 1 cup | 420 | 82 | 4 | 78 | 14 | 2 |
| Plain, cooked | 1 cup | 195 | 40 | 2 | 38 | 7 | 1 |
| **Macaroni & Cheese** | 1 cup | 300 | 40 | 3 | 37 | 10 | 10 |
| **Mackerel** – see Fish | ... | ... | . | . | . | . | . |
| *Malt O Meal*, as prep | 1 cup | 122 | 26 | 1 | 25 | 4 | Tr |
| **Mandarin Oranges** | | | | | | | |
| Canned in light syrup | 1 cup | 154 | 41 | 2 | 39 | 1 | Tr |
| Mango | | | | | | | |
| Fresh, peeled, 11 oz | 1 mango | 135 | 35 | 4 | 31 | 1 | 1 |
| Fresh, peeled, sliced | 1 cup | 105 | 28 | 3 | 25 | 1 | Tr |
| **Manicotti**, 3 cheese | 2 pieces | 300 | 40 | 1 | 39 | 16 | 9 |
| Margarine | | | | | | | |
| **Regular, 4 sticks/Lb** | **1 stick** | **815** | **1** | **0** | **1** | **1** | **90** |
| **Regular, hard or soft** | **1 cup** | **1625** | **1** | **0** | **1** | **2** | **185** |
| **Regular, hard or soft** | **1 Tbsp** | **100** | **Tr** | **0** | **Tr** | **Tr** | **11** |
| **Regular, hard or soft** | **1 tsp** | **34** | **Tr** | **0** | **Tr** | **Tr** | **4** |
| **Reduced fat 50%** | **1 cup** | **1235** | **0** | **0** | **0** | **1** | **139** |
| **Reduced fat 50%** | **1 tsp** | **25** | **0** | **0** | **0** | **Tr** | **3** |
| **Fat free** | **1 cup** | **512** | **0** | **0** | **0** | **Tr** | **Tr** |
| **Fat free** | **1 Tbsp** | **5** | **0** | **0** | **0** | **0** | **0** |
| **Spread or blend type, regular** | **1 Tbsp** | **100** | **Tr** | **0** | **Tr** | **Tr** | **11** |

|  | Serving Size | Calories (g) | Total Carbs(g) | Fiber (g) | Net Carbs(g) | Protein (g) | Fat (g) |
|---|---|---|---|---|---|---|---|
| **Spread or blend w/ vegetable oil & margarine, 33% reduced fat** | **1 Tbsp** | **60** | **0** | **0** | **0** | **0** | **7** |
| **Marjoram, dried spice** | **1 tsp** | **2** | **Tr** | **Tr** | **Tr** | **Tr** | **0** |
| Marmalade | 1 Tbsp | 50 | 14 | Tr | 14 | Tr | Tr |
| Marshmallow |  |  |  |  |  |  |  |
| Miniature size | 1 cup | 160 | 41 | Tr | 41 | Tr | Tr |
| Regular size | 2 piece | 46 | 12 | Tr | 12 | Tr | Tr |
| Regular or Large size | 1 oz | 90 | 23 | Tr | 23 | Tr | Tr |
| Marshmallow Topping | 1 Tbsp | 50 | 12 | Tr | 12 | Tr | Tr |
| Mayonnaise |  |  |  |  |  |  |  |
| **Regular** | **1 Tbsp** | **100** | **Tr** | **0** | **Tr** | **Tr** | **11** |
| **Light / reduced calorie** | **1 Tbsp** | **50** | **1** | **0** | **1** | **Tr** | **5** |
| **Fat free** | **1 Tbsp** | **10** | **2** | **0** | **2** | **Tr** | **0** |
| **Meat** – see specific listings | ... | ... | . | . | . | . | . |
| **Meat Tenderizer** | **1/4 tsp** | **0** | **0** | **0** | **0** | **0** | **0** |
| Meatless Burger |  |  |  |  |  |  |  |
| Single patty, broiled | 1 patty | 100 | 9 | 4 | 5 | 15 | 1 |
| **Cooked, crumbled** | **1 cup** | **230** | **7** | **5** | **2** | **22** | **13** |
| Meatloaf |  |  |  |  |  |  |  |
| *Banquet entrée* | 1 meal | 280 | 22 | 1 | 21 | 13 | 16 |
| *Healthy Choice entrée* | 1 meal | 320 | 52 | 1 | 51 | 15 | 5 |
| *Lean Cuisine entrée* | 1 meal | 260 | 28 | 1 | 27 | 20 | 7 |
| Meatloaf & cheese sandwich | 1 | 350 | 41 | 2 | 39 | 18 | 13 |
| **Minestrone** – see Soup | ... | ... | . | . | . | . | . |
| Molasses, blackstrap | 1 Tbsp | 47 | 12 | 0 | 12 | 0 | 0 |
|  | 1 cup | 771 | 199 | 0 | 199 | 0 | 0 |
| **Mortadella** | **1 slice** | **50** | **Tr** | **0** | **Tr** | **2** | **4** |
| Muffin |  |  |  |  |  |  |  |
| Avg size muffin, 2 ½" dia |  |  |  |  |  |  |  |
| Apple | 1 | 160 | 28 | 2 | 26 | 3 | 4 |
| Banana | 1 | 165 | 29 | 2 | 27 | 3 | 4 |
| Blueberry | 1 | 160 | 28 | 2 | 26 | 3 | 4 |
| Bran w/ raisins | 1 | 175 | 36 | 4 | 32 | 4 | 5 |

| | Serving Size | Calories (g) | Total Carbs(g) | Fiber (g) | Net Carbs(g) | Protein (g) | Fat (g) |
|---|---|---|---|---|---|---|---|
| Chocolate Chip | 1 | 180 | 37 | 2 | 35 | 3 | 5 |
| Corn | 1 | 175 | 29 | 2 | 27 | 3 | 5 |
| Extra large muffin, 4" dia | | | | | | | |
| Banana nut | 1 | 420 | 75 | 8 | 67 | 7 | 11 |
| Bran w/raisins | 1 | 425 | 76 | 8 | 68 | 8 | 11 |
| (also see English Muffin) | | | | | | | |
| *Mulberries* | *½ cup* | *30* | *7* | *3* | *4* | *Tr* | *Tr* |
| Mushroom | | | | | | | |
| Regular Mushrooms | | | | | | | |
| *Fresh, raw, slices* | *1 cup* | *18* | *3* | *1* | *2* | *2* | *Tr* |
| Fresh, sliced, cooked | 1 cup | 42 | 8 | 3 | 5 | 3 | Tr |
| *Canned, stems & pieces, cooked* | *1 cup* | *37* | *8* | *4* | *4* | *3* | *Tr* |
| Shiitake Mushrooms | | | | | | | |
| Dried, cut pieces, cooked | 1 cup | 80 | 20 | 3 | 17 | 2 | Tr |
| *Dried, whole, cooked* | *1 whole* | *11* | *3* | *Tr* | *3* | *Tr* | *Tr* |
| Mussels | | | | | | | |
| – see Fish/Seafood | ... | ... | . | . | . | . | . |
| Mustard, yellow | | | | | | | |
| *Regular* | *1 tsp* | *4* | *Tr* | *Tr* | *Tr* | *Tr* | *Tr* |
| *Hot or Honey flavored* | *1 tsp* | *8* | *2* | *Tr* | *2* | *Tr* | *Tr* |
| *Powder* | *1 tsp* | *10* | *2* | *Tr* | *2* | *Tr* | *Tr* |
| Mustard Greens | | | | | | | |
| *Chopped, cooked* | *1 cup* | *21* | *3* | *2* | *1* | *3* | *Tr* |
| Nachos w/Cheese sauce | 7 pieces | 345 | 36 | 3 | 33 | 9 | 19 |
| Nectarine, fresh, med, 2 ½" dia | 1 | 67 | 16 | 2 | 14 | 1 | 1 |
| Noodles (egg noodles) | | | | | | | |
| Dry, uncooked | 1 cup | 420 | 82 | 4 | 78 | 14 | 2 |
| Plain, cooked | 1 cup | 195 | 40 | 2 | 38 | 7 | 1 |
| Chow Mein noodles, dry crunchy | 1 cup | 235 | 26 | 2 | 24 | 4 | 14 |
| Spinach noodles, cooked | 1 cup | 210 | 39 | 4 | 35 | 8 | 3 |
| Noodles Alfredo | ¾ cup | 250 | 39 | 2 | 37 | 10 | 7 |
| Noodles Stroganoff | ¾ cup | 220 | 37 | 2 | 35 | 9 | 4 |
| Nut Pastry Filling | 1 Tbsp | 65 | 13 | 1 | 12 | 2 | 2 |

| | Serving Size | Calories (g) | Total Carbs(g) | Fiber (g) | Net Carbs(g) | Protein (g) | Fat (g) |
|---|---|---|---|---|---|---|---|
| **Nuts** | | | | | | | |
| Almonds | | | | | | | |
|   sliced almonds | 1 cup | 550 | 19 | 11 | 8 | 20 | 48 |
|   ***whole almonds, about 24*** | *1 oz* | *165* | *6* | *3* | *3* | *6* | *14* |
| ***Brazil nuts, shelled, 6 to 8 nuts*** | *1 oz* | *185* | *4* | *2* | *2* | *4* | *19* |
| Cashews | | | | | | | |
|   dry roasted, about 20 | 1 oz | 160 | 9 | 1 | 8 | 4 | 13 |
|   oil roasted, about 18 | 1 oz | 165 | 8 | 1 | 7 | 5 | 14 |
| Chestnuts, roasted, shelled | 1 cup | 350 | 76 | 7 | 69 | 5 | 3 |
| ***Hazelnuts, chopped, ¼ cup*** | *1 oz* | *180* | *5* | *3* | *2* | *4* | *17* |
| ***Macadamia, dry roasted, 11 nuts*** | *1 oz* | *205* | *4* | *2* | *2* | *2* | *22* |
| Mixed Nuts w/ peanuts | | | | | | | |
|   ***dry roasted, about 20 nuts*** | *1 oz* | *168* | *7* | *3* | *4* | *5* | *15* |
|   ***oil roasted, about 20 nuts*** | *1 oz* | *175* | *6* | *3* | *3* | *5* | *16* |
| Peanuts | | | | | | | |
|   dry roasted, unsalted | 1 cup | 855 | 31 | 12 | 19 | 35 | 73 |
|   ***dry roasted, unsalted, about 28*** | *1 oz* | *165* | *6* | *2* | *4* | *7* | *14* |
|   ***dry roasted, salted, about 28*** | *1 oz* | *165* | *6* | *2* | *4* | *7* | *14* |
|   honey roasted, about 28 | 1 oz | 165 | 7 | 2 | 5 | 7 | 13 |
|   ***oil roasted, salted, about 26*** | *1 oz* | *170* | *5* | *3* | *2* | *7* | *15* |
| ***Pecans, 10 whole or 20 halves*** | *1 oz* | *195* | *4* | *3* | *1* | *3* | *20* |
| ***Pine nuts, shelled*** | *1 oz* | *160* | *4* | *1* | *3* | *7* | *14* |
| Pistachio nuts, dry roasted, shelled, about 47 | 1 oz | 160 | 8 | 3 | 5 | 6 | 13 |
| Walnuts, English | | | | | | | |
|   chopped | 1 cup | 785 | 16 | 8 | 8 | 18 | 78 |
|   ***whole, 7 walnuts*** | *1 oz* | *185* | *4* | *2* | *2* | *4* | *18* |
| **Oat Bran** | | | | | | | |
| Uncooked | 1 cup | 230 | 62 | 15 | 47 | 16 | 7 |
| Cooked | 1 cup | 88 | 25 | 6 | 19 | 7 | 2 |

| | Serving Size | Calories (g) | Total Carbs(g) | Fiber (g) | Net Carbs(g) | Protein (g) | Fat (g) |
|---|---|---|---|---|---|---|---|
| **Oatmeal**, as prep | | | | | | | |
| Plain, sweetened | ½ cup | 75 | 13 | 2 | 11 | 3 | 1 |
| Fruit flavored oatmeal | 1 pkt | 135 | 26 | 2 | 24 | 3 | 2 |
| Maple & brown | | | | | | | |
| sugar oatmeal | 1 pkt | 130 | 27 | 6 | 21 | 3 | 1 |
| **Oats**, dry, 100% rolled oats | ½ cup | 150 | 26 | 4 | 22 | 5 | 3 |
| **OIL** (for cooking & salads) | | | | | | | |
| *Cooking spray,* | | | | | | | |
| *¼ second spray* | *1 spray* | *0* | *0* | *0* | *0* | *0* | *0* |
| *Canola oil* | *1 cup* | *1925* | *0* | *0* | *0* | *0* | *218* |
| *Canola oil* | *Tbsp* | *120* | *0* | *0* | *0* | *0* | *14* |
| *Corn oil* | *1 cup* | *1925* | *0* | *0* | *0* | *0* | *218* |
| *Corn oil* | *Tbsp* | *120* | *0* | *0* | *0* | *0* | *14* |
| *Cottonseed/soybean* | | | | | | | |
| *oil blend* | *1 cup* | *1925* | *0* | *0* | *0* | *0* | *218* |
| *Cottonseed/soybean* | | | | | | | |
| *oil blend* | *1 Tbsp* | *120* | *0* | *0* | *0* | *0* | *14* |
| *Olive oil* | *1 cup* | *1905* | *0* | *0* | *0* | *0* | *216* |
| *Olive oil* | *1 Tbsp* | *119* | *0* | *0* | *0* | *0* | *14* |
| *Peanut oil* | *1 cup* | *1905* | *0* | *0* | *0* | *0* | *216* |
| *Peanut oil* | *1 Tbsp* | *119* | *0* | *0* | *0* | *0* | *14* |
| *Safflower oil* | *1 cup* | *1925* | *0* | *0* | *0* | *0* | *218* |
| *Safflower oil* | *1 Tbsp* | *120* | *0* | *0* | *0* | *0* | *14* |
| *Sesame oil* | *1 cup* | *1925* | *0* | *0* | *0* | *0* | *218* |
| *Sesame oil* | *1 Tbsp* | *120* | *0* | *0* | *0* | *0* | *14* |
| *Soybean oil* | *1 cup* | *1925* | *0* | *0* | *0* | *0* | *218* |
| *Soybean oil* | *1 Tbsp* | *120* | *0* | *0* | *0* | *0* | *14* |
| *Sunflower oil* | *1 cup* | *1925* | *0* | *0* | *0* | *0* | *218* |
| *Sunflower oil* | *1 Tbsp* | *120* | *0* | *0* | *0* | *0* | *14* |
| *Vegetable oil* | *1 cup* | *1925* | *0* | *0* | *0* | *0* | *218* |
| *Vegetable oil* | *1 Tbsp* | *120* | *0* | *0* | *0* | *0* | *14* |
| **Okra** | | | | | | | |
| Fresh, sliced, cooked | 1 cup | 51 | 12 | 4 | 8 | 3 | Tr |
| Frozen, slices, cooked | 1 cup | 52 | 11 | 5 | 6 | 4 | 1 |
| Whole, 3" pods, cooked | 8 pods | 30 | 7 | 2 | 5 | 2 | Tr |
| Fried, breaded | ½ cup | 165 | 17 | 4 | 13 | 3 | 10 |
| **Olive** | | | | | | | |
| *Pickled, green,* | | | | | | | |
| *med size* | *5* | *20* | *Tr* | *Tr* | *Tr* | *Tr* | *2* |
| *Ripe, black, Lg size* | *5* | *25* | *1* | *Tr* | *Tr* | *Tr* | *2* |

| | Serving Size | Calories (g) | Total Carbs(g) | Fiber (g) | Net Carbs(g) | Protein (g) | Fat (g) |
|---|---|---|---|---|---|---|---|
| *Olive Loaf* | *2 oz* | *130* | *1* | *Tr* | *Tr* | *6* | *12* |
| Onion | | | | | | | |
| Round yellow or white onion | | | | | | | |
| Fresh, raw, whole, 2 ½" dia | 1 whole | 42 | 9 | 2 | 7 | 1 | Tr |
| Fresh, chopped | 1 cup | 61 | 14 | 3 | 11 | 2 | Tr |
| *Fresh, sliced, ⅛" thick* | *1 slice* | *5* | *1* | *Tr* | *Tr* | *Tr* | *Tr* |
| Cooked, whole, 2 ½" dia | 1 whole | 41 | 10 | 1 | 9 | 1 | Tr |
| Cooked, sliced or chopped | 1 cup | 92 | 21 | 3 | 18 | 3 | Tr |
| Sprigs w/green tops & bulbs | | | | | | | |
| *Whole w/top, raw, chopped* | *1 whole* | *8* | *1* | *Tr* | *Tr* | *1* | *Tr* |
| *Bulbs only, chopped* | *1 cup* | *32* | *7* | *3* | *4* | *2* | *Tr* |
| *Onion Flakes, dried* | *1 Tbsp* | *16* | *4* | *Tr* | *4* | *Tr* | *Tr* |
| *Onion Powder or Salt* | *1 tsp* | *7* | *2* | *Tr* | *2* | *Tr* | *Tr* |
| Onion Rings | | | | | | | |
| Breaded, fried | 5 rings | 125 | 13 | 1 | 12 | 2 | 7 |
| Orange | | | | | | | |
| Fresh, medium size, 3" dia | 1 | 70 | 15 | 3 | 12 | 1 | Tr |
| Fresh, sections | 1 cup | 85 | 20 | 4 | 16 | 2 | Tr |
| *Oregano, ground* | *1 tsp* | *5* | *1* | *Tr* | *Tr* | *Tr* | *Tr* |
| *Pam,* non-stick cooking spray | | | | | | | |
| *¼ second spray* | *1 spray* | *0* | *0* | *0* | *0* | *0* | *0* |
| Pancake, 4" dia | | | | | | | |
| Regular, toaster type | 1 | 82 | 16 | 1 | 15 | 2 | 1 |
| Lowfat, toaster type | 1 | 70 | 17 | 1 | 16 | 2 | Tr |
| Regular, from mix or scratch | 1 | 90 | 17 | 1 | 16 | 2 | 2 |
| Blueberry, mix or toaster type | 1 | 85 | 15 | 1 | 14 | 2 | 1 |
| Pancake Syrup – see Syrup | ... | ... | . | . | . | . | . |
| Papaya | | | | | | | |
| Fresh, peeled, 5" long x 3" dia | 1 | 120 | 30 | 6 | 24 | 2 | Tr |

| | Serving Size | Calories (g) | Total Carbs(g) | Fiber (g) | Net Carbs(g) | Protein (g) | Fat (g) |
|---|---|---|---|---|---|---|---|
| Fresh, peeled, cubed | 1 cup | 55 | 14 | 3 | 11 | 1 | Tr |
| *Paprika, dried powder* | *1 tsp* | *6* | *1* | *Tr* | *Tr* | *Tr* | *Tr* |
| Parsley | | | | | | | |
| *Fresh, raw, chopped* | *10 sprigs* | *4* | *1* | *Tr* | *Tr* | *Tr* | *Tr* |
| *Dried parsley bits* | *1 Tbsp* | *4* | *1* | *Tr* | *Tr* | *Tr* | *Tr* |
| Parsnip, sliced, cooked | 1 cup | 125 | 30 | 6 | 24 | 2 | Tr |
| *Passion Fruit, raw, avg size* | *1* | *17* | *4* | *Tr* | *4* | *Tr* | *Tr* |
| Pasta | | | | | | | |
| Plain, cooked | 1 cup | 195 | 40 | 2 | 38 | 7 | 1 |
| W/cheese & tomato sauce | 1 cup | 250 | 41 | 3 | 38 | 7 | 6 |
| W/meatballs in tomato sauce | 1 cup | 260 | 31 | 3 | 28 | 11 | 10 |
| W/shrimp & herb sauce | 1 cup | 295 | 40 | 3 | 37 | 10 | 10 |
| W/tomato sauce | 1 cup | 240 | 41 | 3 | 38 | 7 | 5 |
| *Pasta Roni* | | | | | | | |
| Pasta w/broccoli | 1 cup | 240 | 37 | 3 | 34 | 7 | 4 |
| Pasta w/broccoli & chicken | 1 cup | 260 | 37 | 3 | 34 | 8 | 5 |
| **Pasta Alfredo Primavera** | 1 cup | 280 | 44 | 3 | 41 | 11 | 7 |
| **Pasta, Angel Hair** | | | | | | | |
| Prep w/herb sauce | 1 cup | 280 | 42 | 3 | 39 | 7 | 9 |
| *Weight Watchers entrée* | 1 meal | 170 | 29 | 2 | 27 | 8 | 2 |
| **Pasta, Bowtie** | | | | | | | |
| w/tomato sauce | 1 cup | 240 | 41 | 3 | 38 | 7 | 5 |
| **Pasta Marsala** | 1 cup | 280 | 36 | 3 | 33 | 13 | 9 |
| **Pasta Salad** w/dressing | 1 cup | 250 | 32 | 2 | 30 | 5 | 10 |
| Pastrami | | | | | | | |
| *Regular* | *2 oz* | *90* | *2* | *Tr* | *2* | *12* | *4* |
| *Turkey* | *2 oz* | *60* | *1* | *Tr* | *Tr* | *13* | *1* |
| **Pastry** – see Danish Pastry & specific listings | ... | ... | . | . | . | . | . |
| **Pastry Filling** – see specific listing | ... | ... | . | . | . | . | . |
| Peach | | | | | | | |
| Fresh, whole, med, 2 ½" dia | 1 | 42 | 11 | 2 | 9 | 1 | Tr |

| | Serving Size | Calories (g) | Total Carbs(g) | Fiber (g) | Net Carbs(g) | Protein (g) | Fat (g) |
|---|---|---|---|---|---|---|---|
| Fresh, sliced | 1 cup | 76 | 19 | 3 | 16 | 1 | Tr |
| Canned, in heavy syrup | 1 cup | 195 | 52 | 3 | 49 | 1 | Tr |
| Canned, in light syrup | 1 cup | 150 | 39 | 2 | 37 | 1 | Tr |
| Canned, in juice | 1 cup | 115 | 28 | 3 | 25 | 2 | Tr |
| Dried, halves, | 3 halves | 93 | 24 | 3 | 21 | 1 | Tr |
| Frozen, sweetened slices, thawed | 1 cup | 235 | 60 | 5 | 55 | 2 | Tr |
| **Peanut** – see Nuts | ... | ... | . | . | . | . | . |
| **Peanut Butter** | | | | | | | |
| *Regular, smooth* | *1 Tbsp* | *95* | *3* | *1* | *2* | *4* | *8* |
| *Regular, chunky* | *1 Tbsp* | *95* | *3* | *1* | *2* | *4* | *8* |
| Reduced fat, smooth | 1 Tbsp | 90 | 6 | 1 | 5 | 5 | 6 |
| **Pear** | | | | | | | |
| Fresh, 2 ½" dia | 1 | 50 | 13 | 4 | 9 | 1 | Tr |
| Fresh, 3 ¼" dia | 1 | 116 | 29 | 9 | 20 | 1 | 1 |
| Canned, in heavy syrup | 1 cup | 197 | 51 | 4 | 47 | 1 | Tr |
| Canned, in juice | 1 cup | 125 | 32 | 4 | 28 | 1 | Tr |
| **Peas** (cooked w/o fats) | | | | | | | |
| Black eyed peas | ½ cup | 105 | 26 | 8 | 18 | 4 | Tr |
| Chickpeas | ½ cup | 140 | 25 | 6 | 19 | 7 | 2 |
| Green peas | ½ cup | 60 | 11 | 4 | 7 | 4 | Tr |
| Lentils | ½ cup | 115 | 20 | 8 | 12 | 9 | 1 |
| Navy peas | ½ cup | 125 | 24 | 6 | 18 | 8 | 1 |
| Pea Pods | ½ cup | 40 | 7 | 2 | 5 | 3 | Tr |
| Split peas | ½ cup | 115 | 20 | 8 | 12 | 8 | 1 |
| Sweet peas | ½ cup | 60 | 11 | 4 | 7 | 4 | Tr |
| **Peas and Carrots** | ½ cup | 40 | 8 | 3 | 5 | 3 | Tr |
| **Pecan Pastry Filling** | 1 Tbsp | 65 | 13 | 1 | 12 | 2 | 2 |
| **Pecans, 10 whole or 20 halves** | *1 oz* | *195* | *4* | *3* | *1* | *3* | *20* |
| **Pepper,** dried powder or granules | | | | | | | |
| *Black* | *1 tsp* | *5* | *1* | *Tr* | *Tr* | *Tr* | *Tr* |
| *Cayenne or red* | *1 tsp* | *7* | *1* | *Tr* | *Tr* | *Tr* | *Tr* |
| *White* | *1 tsp* | *5* | *1* | *Tr* | *Tr* | *Tr* | *Tr* |
| **Pepper Steak** | | | | | | | |
| *Stouffer's entree* | 1 meal | 330 | 45 | 1 | 44 | 17 | 9 |
| *Le Menu entree* | 1 meal | 354 | 35 | 1 | 34 | 26 | 13 |

| | Serving Size | Calories (g) | Total Carbs(g) | Fiber (g) | Net Carbs(g) | Protein (g) | Fat (g) |
|---|---|---|---|---|---|---|---|
| ***Pepperoni,*** | | | | | | | |
| **14 thin slices/oz** | **1 oz** | **130** | **0** | **0** | **0** | **6** | **12** |
| Peppers | | | | | | | |
| Chili Peppers, hot, raw | | | | | | | |
| **red or green** | **1 whole** | **18** | **4** | **1** | **3** | **1** | **Tr** |
| Green, sweet, raw | | | | | | | |
| whole, 3" x 2 ¼" | 1 whole | 32 | 8 | 2 | 6 | 1 | Tr |
| **ring, ¼" thick** | **1 ring** | **3** | **1** | **Tr** | **Tr** | **Tr** | **Tr** |
| chopped | 1 cup | 40 | 10 | 3 | 7 | 1 | Tr |
| **Jalapeno peppers,** | | | | | | | |
| **sliced** | **¼ cup** | **7** | **1** | **Tr** | **Tr** | **Tr** | **Tr** |
| Red, sweet, raw | | | | | | | |
| whole, 3" x 2 ¼" | 1 whole | 32 | 8 | 2 | 6 | 1 | Tr |
| **ring, ¼" thick** | **1 ring** | **3** | **1** | **Tr** | **Tr** | **Tr** | **Tr** |
| chopped | 1 cup | 40 | 10 | 3 | 7 | 1 | Tr |
| Red or Green, | | | | | | | |
| sweet, cooked | | | | | | | |
| chopped | 1 cup | 38 | 9 | 2 | 7 | 1 | Tr |
| **Peppers, Stuffed,** *Stouffers* | 1 cup | 200 | 27 | 3 | 24 | 11 | 5 |
| **Persimmon,** raw, | | | | | | | |
| medium size | 1 | 32 | 8 | 2 | 6 | Tr | Tr |
| Pickle | | | | | | | |
| Bread & Butter | | | | | | | |
| slices, 1 ½" dia | 6 slices | 36 | 8 | 1 | 7 | Tr | Tr |
| **Dill, whole, 3 ¾" long** | **1** | **12** | **3** | **1** | **2** | **Tr** | **Tr** |
| Sweet Gherkin, 2 ½" long | 1 | 20 | 5 | Tr | 5 | Tr | Tr |
| **Pickle Relish** | 1 Tbsp | 20 | 5 | Tr | 5 | Tr | Tr |
| Pie | | | | | | | |
| *(⅛ of 9" pie unless noted)* | | | | | | | |
| Apple pie, 2 crust | 1 slice | 420 | 59 | 4 | 55 | 4 | 19 |
| Blueberry pie, 2 crust | 1 slice | 360 | 49 | 4 | 45 | 4 | 17 |
| Boston Cream Pie, 1 crust | 1 slice | 230 | 39 | 1 | 38 | 2 | 8 |
| Cherry pie, 2 crust | 1 slice | 485 | 69 | 4 | 65 | 5 | 22 |
| Cherry, fried pie, 4" x 2" | 1 slice | 405 | 55 | 3 | 52 | 4 | 21 |
| Chocolate chip pie, 1 crust | 1 slice | 590 | 57 | 3 | 54 | 6 | 34 |
| Chocolate Cream pie, | | | | | | | |
| 1 crust | 1 slice | 405 | 45 | 3 | 42 | 4 | 22 |
| Coconut Custard pie, | | | | | | | |
| 1 crust | 1 slice | 305 | 36 | 2 | 34 | 7 | 15 |

| | Serving Size | Calories (g) | Total Carbs(g) | Fiber (g) | Net Carbs(g) | Protein (g) | Fat (g) |
|---|---|---|---|---|---|---|---|
| Lemon Meringue pie, 1 crust | 1 slice | 360 | 50 | 1 | 49 | 5 | 16 |
| Peach pie, 2 crust | 1 slice | 410 | 58 | 3 | 55 | 4 | 19 |
| Pecan pie, 1 crust | 1 slice | 505 | 64 | 2 | 62 | 6 | 27 |
| Pumpkin pie, 1 crust | 1 slice | 320 | 41 | 3 | 38 | 7 | 14 |
| Strawberry pie, 2 crust | 1 slice | 360 | 50 | 2 | 48 | 5 | 16 |
| **Pie Crust, 9" dia** | | | | | | | |
| Regular from recipe or frozen | 1 crust | 800 | 75 | 2 | 73 | 9 | 50 |
| Graham cracker crust | 1 crust | 950 | 110 | 3 | 107 | 9 | 51 |
| Reduced fat crust | 1 crust | 605 | 74 | 2 | 72 | 8 | 30 |
| **Pilaf** – see Rice Pilaf | ... | ... | . | . | . | . | . |
| *Pimiento* | *1 oz* | *10* | *2* | *Tr* | *2* | *Tr* | *Tr* |
| **Pineapple** | | | | | | | |
| Fresh, diced or sliced | 1 cup | 76 | 19 | 2 | 17 | 1 | 1 |
| Canned, in heavy syrup, | | | | | | | |
| chunks or crushed | 1 cup | 198 | 51 | 2 | 49 | 1 | Tr |
| slices, 3" dia | 1 slice | 38 | 10 | Tr | 10 | Tr | Tr |
| Canned, in juice, | | | | | | | |
| chunks or crushed | 1 cup | 150 | 39 | 2 | 37 | 1 | Tr |
| slices, 3" dia | 1 slice | 28 | 7 | 1 | 6 | Tr | Tr |
| **PIZZA** | | | | | | | |
| *(Listings for an avg size slice, ⅛ of 12" pizza)* | | | | | | | |
| **Thin & Crispy Pizza** | | | | | | | |
| Cheese | 1 slice | 140 | 21 | 1 | 20 | 8 | 3 |
| Pepperoni & Cheese | 1 slice | 180 | 20 | 1 | 19 | 10 | 7 |
| One Meat w/ Vegetables | 1 slice | 185 | 21 | 2 | 19 | 13 | 5 |
| Three Meat w/ Vegetables | 1 slice | 210 | 21 | 2 | 19 | 12 | 9 |
| **Thick & Chewy or Pan Pizza** | | | | | | | |
| Cheese | 1 slice | 270 | 39 | 1 | 38 | 15 | 6 |
| Pepperoni & Cheese | 1 slice | 310 | 39 | 1 | 38 | 19 | 8 |
| One Meat w/ Vegetables | 1 slice | 320 | 38 | 2 | 36 | 15 | 12 |
| Three Meat w/ Vegetables | 1 slice | 405 | 40 | 2 | 38 | 24 | 17 |

| | Serving Size | Calories (g) | Total Carbs(g) | Fiber (g) | Net Carbs(g) | Protein (g) | Fat (g) |
|---|---|---|---|---|---|---|---|
| **Stuffed Crust Pizza,** thick | | | | | | | |
| Pepperoni & Cheese | 1 slice | 350 | 39 | 1 | 38 | 20 | 14 |
| Three Meat w/ Vegetables | 1 slice | 450 | 40 | 2 | 38 | 21 | 21 |
| **Pizza Rolls,** 1 ½", frozen, heated | | | | | | | |
| w/ cheese and one meat | 5 pieces | 175 | 20 | 1 | 19 | 9 | 7 |
| **Plantain,** without peel | | | | | | | |
| Fresh, medium size | 1 | 218 | 57 | 4 | 53 | 2 | 1 |
| Cooked, slices | 1 cup | 180 | 48 | 4 | 44 | 1 | Tr |
| **Plum** | | | | | | | |
| Fresh, whole, med, 2 ¼" dia | 1 | 36 | 9 | 1 | 8 | 1 | Tr |
| Canned, in heavy syrup | 1 cup | 230 | 60 | 3 | 57 | 1 | Tr |
| Canned, in juice | 1 cup | 146 | 38 | 3 | 35 | 1 | Tr |
| **Pomegranate,** avg size, raw | 1 | 105 | 26 | 2 | 24 | 2 | 1 |
| **Pop Tart** – see Toaster Pastry | ... | ... | . | . | . | . | . |
| **Popcorn** | | | | | | | |
| Air popped | 1 cup | 30 | 6 | 1 | 5 | 1 | Tr |
| Caramel coated w/ peanuts | 1 cup | 170 | 34 | 2 | 32 | 3 | 3 |
| Caramel coated w/o peanuts | 1 cup | 150 | 28 | 2 | 26 | 1 | 5 |
| Cheese flavored | 1 cup | 60 | 6 | 1 | 5 | 1 | 4 |
| *Microwave, butter flavor* | *1 cup* | *40* | *4* | *1* | *3* | *1* | *2* |
| Microwave, butter, *reduced fat* | *1 cup* | *30* | *5* | *1* | *4* | *1* | *1* |
| Popped in oil | 1 cup | 55 | 6 | 1 | 5 | 1 | 3 |
| Popped in oil, buttered | 1 cup | 75 | 6 | 1 | 5 | 1 | 5 |
| **Popcorn Cake,** plain | 1 | 38 | 8 | Tr | 8 | 1 | Tr |
| Butter flavor | 1 | 40 | 8 | Tr | 8 | 1 | Tr |
| Carmel | 1 | 48 | 11 | Tr | 11 | 1 | Tr |
| **Poppyseed pastry filling** | 1 Tbsp | 65 | 14 | 1 | 13 | 1 | 1 |
| **Popsicle** – see Frozen Dessert | ... | ... | . | . | . | . | . |

| | Serving Size | Calories (g) | Total Carbs(g) | Fiber (g) | Net Carbs(g) | Protein (g) | Fat (g) |
|---|---|---|---|---|---|---|---|
| **PORK** | | | | | | | |
| *(Weights for meat w/o bones)* | | | | | | | |
| **Bacon, regular** | **3 slices** | **110** | **Tr** | **0** | **Tr** | **6** | **9** |
| **Bacon, Canadian** | **3 slices** | **125** | **1** | **0** | **1** | **17** | **6** |
| **Boston Butt, roasted, lean** | **3 oz** | **205** | **0** | **0** | **0** | **27** | **9** |
| **Picnic Pork** | **3.5 oz** | **280** | **Tr** | **0** | **Tr** | **20** | **21** |
| **Pork Chop, loin cut** | | | | | | | |
| **broiled, lean & fat** | **3 oz** | **205** | **0** | **0** | **0** | **24** | **11** |
| **broiled, lean only** | **3 oz** | **170** | **0** | **0** | **0** | **26** | **7** |
| **pan fried, lean & fat** | **3 oz** | **235** | **0** | **0** | **0** | **25** | **14** |
| **pan fried, lean only** | **3 oz** | **195** | **0** | **0** | **0** | **27** | **9** |
| **Rib Roast, lean & fat** | **3 oz** | **215** | **0** | **0** | **0** | **23** | **13** |
| **lean only** | **3 oz** | **195** | **0** | **0** | **0** | **24** | **9** |
| Sausage | | | | | | | |
| **breakfast link, small** | **1 link** | **70** | **Tr** | **0** | **Tr** | **3** | **6** |
| **breakfast patty, small** | **1 patty** | **80** | **Tr** | **0** | **Tr** | **3** | **7** |
| **sausage, regular** | **2 oz** | **120** | **1** | **0** | **1** | **7** | **10** |
| sausage, lowfat | 2 oz | 80 | 6 | 0 | 6 | 7 | 2 |
| **Polish Kielbasa sausage** | **2 oz** | **120** | **Tr** | **0** | **Tr** | **8** | **10** |
| **Vienna sausage, 2" links** | **2 links** | **90** | **Tr** | **0** | **Tr** | **4** | **8** |
| **Shoulder cut, braised, lean & fat** | **3 oz** | **280** | **0** | **0** | **0** | **24** | **20** |
| **lean only** | **3 oz** | **210** | **0** | **0** | **0** | **27** | **10** |
| **Spareribs, braised** | **3 oz** | **335** | **0** | **0** | **0** | **25** | **26** |
| (Other Pork Products, see: Bologna, Ham, Hot Dog, Salami, & specific entrées) | ... | ... | . | . | . | . | . |
| **Pork Chop,** fried | | | | | | | |
| Marie Callender entrée | 1 meal | 550 | 50 | 2 | 48 | 26 | 27 |
| **Pork Rinds, about 1 cup** | **1 oz** | **155** | **0** | **0** | **0** | **17** | **9** |
| Pot Pie, 4" dia, frozen, heated | | | | | | | |
| Beef Pot Pie | 1 pie | 480 | 40 | 2 | 38 | 19 | 27 |
| Chicken Pot Pie | 1 pie | 410 | 38 | 2 | 36 | 11 | 23 |
| Turkey Pot Pie | 1 pie | 400 | 38 | 2 | 36 | 11 | 22 |

| | Serving Size | Calories (g) | Total Carbs(g) | Fiber (g) | Net Carbs(g) | Protein (g) | Fat (g) |
|---|---|---|---|---|---|---|---|
| **Pot Roast** | | | | | | | |
| Lean Cuisine entrée | 1 meal | 190 | 19 | 1 | 18 | 15 | 6 |
| Marie Callender entrée | 1 meal | 250 | 31 | 1 | 30 | 17 | 6 |
| Swanson entrée | 1 meal | 405 | 48 | 2 | 46 | 30 | 10 |
| **POTATO** | | | | | | | |
| *(also see Sweet Potatoes)* | | | | | | | |
| Au Gratin Potatoes | 1 cup | 300 | 28 | 4 | 24 | 9 | 16 |
| Baked potato, 4 ¾" x 2 ¼" | | | | | | | |
| whole potato w/skin | 1 | 220 | 51 | 5 | 46 | 5 | Tr |
| whole potato w/o skin | 1 | 145 | 34 | 2 | 32 | 3 | Tr |
| Baked, & filled or topped, large potato, 6" x 2 ½" | | | | | | | |
| bacon & cheese | 1 | 530 | 78 | 5 | 73 | 17 | 18 |
| broccoli & cheese | 1 | 470 | 80 | 6 | 74 | 9 | 14 |
| cheese | 1 | 570 | 78 | 5 | 73 | 14 | 23 |
| chili & cheese | 1 | 620 | 83 | 5 | 78 | 20 | 24 |
| sour cream & chives | 1 | 390 | 73 | 6 | 67 | 7 | 6 |
| Boiled potato, 2 ½" dia | | | | | | | |
| peeled, whole potato | 1 | 116 | 27 | 2 | 25 | 2 | Tr |
| peeled, diced | 1 cup | 134 | 31 | 3 | 28 | 3 | Tr |
| French Fries | | | | | | | |
| Frozen, heated | | | | | | | |
| thin shoestring strips, 3 oz | 20 fries | 130 | 22 | 2 | 20 | 2 | 4 |
| thick or crinkle cut, 4.5 oz | 20 fries | 195 | 33 | 3 | 30 | 3 | 6 |
| Restaurant type, medium order | 1 med | 350 | 48 | 5 | 43 | 5 | 15 |
| Hash Browns, patty, 3" x 2" | 1 patty | 80 | 9 | 1 | 8 | 2 | 9 |
| Hash Browned potatoes | 1 cup | 280 | 32 | 2 | 30 | 4 | 14 |
| Mashed, w/milk & margarine | 1 cup | 220 | 35 | 4 | 31 | 4 | 9 |
| Scalloped potatoes | 1 cup | 245 | 29 | 4 | 25 | 8 | 11 |
| Tater Tots type fried potatoes | 10 | 175 | 24 | 3 | 21 | 3 | 8 |
| **Potato Chips** | | | | | | | |
| *(about 14 chips, unless noted)* | | | | | | | |
| Plain, regular | 1 oz | 155 | 15 | 1 | 14 | 2 | 10 |
| Barbecue flavor | 1 oz | 155 | 15 | 1 | 14 | 2 | 10 |

| | Serving Size | Calories (g) | Total Carbs(g) | Fiber (g) | Net Carbs(g) | Protein (g) | Fat (g) |
|---|---|---|---|---|---|---|---|
| Cheddar cheese | 1 oz | 160 | 15 | 1 | 14 | 2 | 10 |
| Fat free chips | 1 oz | 75 | 17 | 1 | 16 | 2 | Tr |
| *Pringles*, regular | 1 oz | 160 | 15 | 1 | 14 | 1 | 11 |
| Reduced fat chips | 1 oz | 140 | 18 | 1 | 17 | 2 | 7 |
| Rippled chips | | | | | | | |
| (about 12 chips) | 1 oz | 160 | 15 | 1 | 14 | 2 | 10 |
| *Ruffles*, original (12 chips) | 1 oz | 160 | 14 | 1 | 13 | 2 | 10 |
| *Ruffles*, reduced fat | | | | | | | |
| (13 chips) | 1 oz | 150 | 18 | 1 | 17 | 2 | 7 |
| Ranch flavor chips | 1 oz | 155 | 15 | 2 | 13 | 2 | 10 |
| Sour cream & onion flavor | 1 oz | 155 | 15 | 2 | 13 | 2 | 10 |
| **Potato Salad** | 1 cup | 360 | 28 | 3 | 25 | 7 | 21 |
| **Potato Sticks,** | | | | | | | |
| fried, crunchy | 1 cup | 250 | 26 | 3 | 23 | 3 | 15 |
| **Preserves** | | | | | | | |
| All flavors, regular | 1 Tbsp | 55 | 14 | Tr | 14 | Tr | Tr |
| All flavors, restaurant | | | | | | | |
| packet | 1 pkt | 39 | 10 | Tr | 10 | Tr | Tr |
| **Pretzels** | | | | | | | |
| Sticks, regular | 25 | 58 | 12 | 1 | 11 | 1 | 1 |
| Mini Twists, regular | 10 | 58 | 12 | 1 | 11 | 1 | 1 |
| Bavarian, twisted, | | | | | | | |
| 2 ½" x 3" | 1 | 60 | 13 | 1 | 12 | 1 | 1 |
| Chocolate coated | 1 oz | 130 | 20 | 1 | 19 | 2 | 5 |
| Dutch, twisted, 2 ½" x 3" | 1 | 60 | 13 | 1 | 12 | 1 | 1 |
| Honey Mustard nuggets | 10 | 150 | 24 | 1 | 23 | 3 | 4 |
| Soft, twisted, large, | | | | | | | |
| 3" x 5" | 1 | 180 | 36 | 2 | 34 | 5 | 2 |
| Sourdough, twisted, | | | | | | | |
| 2 ½" x 3" | 1 | 60 | 13 | 1 | 12 | 1 | 1 |
| ***Prosciutto, Boars Head*** | ***1 oz*** | ***60*** | ***0*** | ***0*** | ***0*** | ***8*** | ***3*** |
| **Prunes,** dried, pitted | 5 prunes | 100 | 26 | 3 | 23 | 1 | Tr |
| Uncooked, unsweetened | | | | | | | |
| Stewed, unsweetened | 1 cup | 265 | 70 | 16 | 54 | 3 | 1 |
| **Pudding** | | | | | | | |
| Butterscotch, regular | ½ cup | 150 | 25 | Tr | 25 | 3 | 5 |
| Caramel w/chocolate, | | | | | | | |
| regular | ½ cup | 150 | 25 | 1 | 24 | 3 | 5 |

| | Serving Size | Calories (g) | Total Carbs(g) | Fiber (g) | Net Carbs(g) | Protein (g) | Fat (g) |
|---|---|---|---|---|---|---|---|
| Chocolate, regular | ½ cup | 150 | 25 | 1 | 24 | 3 | 5 |
| fat free | ½ cup | 105 | 23 | 1 | 22 | 3 | Tr |
| sugar free | ½ cup | 110 | 18 | 1 | 17 | 2 | 1 |
| Rice pudding, regular | ½ cup | 185 | 25 | Tr | 25 | 2 | 8 |
| Tapioca, regular | ½ cup | 135 | 22 | Tr | 22 | 2 | 4 |
| fat free | ½ cup | 100 | 23 | Tr | 23 | 2 | Tr |
| Vanilla, regular | ½ cup | 145 | 25 | Tr | 25 | 3 | 4 |
| fat free | ½ cup | 105 | 24 | Tr | 24 | 2 | Tr |
| sugar free | ½ cup | 110 | 18 | Tr | 18 | 2 | 1 |
| **Pumpkin** | | | | | | | |
| Fresh, cooked, mashed | 1 cup | 50 | 12 | 3 | 9 | 2 | Tr |
| Canned, heated | 1 cup | 83 | 20 | 7 | 13 | 3 | 1 |
| **Quesadilla** | | | | | | | |
| Cheese | 1 | 350 | 31 | 2 | 29 | 16 | 18 |
| Chicken | 1 | 400 | 33 | 2 | 31 | 25 | 19 |
| ***Radish, fresh, raw, avg 1" dia*** | *5* | *5* | *1* | *Tr* | *Tr* | *Tr* | *Tr* |
| **Raisin** | | | | | | | |
| Golden or natural, not packed | 1 cup | 435 | 115 | 6 | 109 | 5 | 1 |
| Golden or natural, 0.5 oz pkg | 1 pkg | 42 | 11 | 1 | 10 | Tr | Tr |
| Golden or natural, not packed | 3 Tbsp | 84 | 22 | 1 | 21 | Tr | Tr |
| **Raisin Bran** – see Cereal | | | | | | | |
| **Raspberries** | | | | | | | |
| Fresh | 1 cup | 60 | 14 | 8 | 6 | 1 | 1 |
| Frozen, sweetened, thawed | 1 cup | 260 | 65 | 11 | 54 | 2 | Tr |
| **Ravioli** | | | | | | | |
| Beef | 1 cup | 255 | 44 | 1 | 43 | 12 | 4 |
| Cheese | 1 cup | 265 | 44 | 1 | 43 | 11 | 5 |
| **Relish** – see Pickle Relish or specific listing | ... | ... | . | . | . | . | . |
| **Rhubarb** | | | | | | | |
| Fresh, diced | 1 cup | 28 | 6 | Tr | 6 | Tr | Tr |
| Frozen, cooked, sweetened | 1 cup | 278 | 75 | 5 | 70 | 1 | Tr |

| | Serving Size | Calories (g) | Total Carbs(g) | Fiber (g) | Net Carbs(g) | Protein (g) | Fat (g) |
|---|---|---|---|---|---|---|---|
| **RICE** | | | | | | | |
| **Plain Rice Dishes** | | | | | | | |
| Brown long grain rice, boiled | 1 cup | 215 | 45 | 4 | 41 | 5 | 2 |
| Brown long grain, prep w/butter | 1 cup | 315 | 45 | 4 | 41 | 5 | 13 |
| Long grain & wild rice, boiled | 1 cup | 200 | 40 | 3 | 37 | 6 | 1 |
| Long grain & wild prep w/butter | 1 cup | 300 | 40 | 3 | 37 | 6 | 12 |
| White rice, boiled | 1 cup | 200 | 44 | 1 | 43 | 4 | Tr |
| White rice, prep w/butter | 1 cup | 300 | 44 | 1 | 43 | 4 | 11 |
| Wild rice, boiled | 1 cup | 170 | 35 | 3 | 32 | 7 | 1 |
| Wild rice, prep w/butter | 1 cup | 270 | 35 | 3 | 32 | 7 | 12 |
| Yellow rice, boiled | 1 cup | 220 | 49 | 3 | 46 | 5 | Tr |
| **Mixed & Flavored** | | | | | | | |
| **Rice Dishes** | | | | | | | |
| Flavored w/ beef or pork | 1 cup | 280 | 52 | 3 | 49 | 8 | 4 |
| Fried rice w/ beef | 1 cup | 295 | 48 | 3 | 45 | 10 | 7 |
| Fried rice w/ chicken | 1 cup | 265 | 44 | 3 | 41 | 9 | 6 |
| Fried rice w/ pork | 1 cup | 290 | 48 | 3 | 45 | 11 | 6 |
| Fried rice w/ shrimp | 1 cup | 260 | 44 | 3 | 41 | 9 | 5 |
| Fried rice w/ vegetables | 1 cup | 255 | 48 | 3 | 45 | 7 | 4 |
| Rice & beans | 1 cup | 300 | 49 | 3 | 46 | 11 | 7 |
| Rice & vegetables | 1 cup | 260 | 50 | 3 | 47 | 8 | 3 |
| Rice Pilaf w/vegetables | 1 cup | 240 | 45 | 3 | 42 | 6 | 3 |
| **Rice-a-Roni** | | | | | | | |
| Beef vermicelli rice dish | 1 cup | 290 | 51 | 3 | 48 | 9 | 4 |
| Broccoli & cheddar rice dish | 1 cup | 330 | 48 | 3 | 45 | 10 | 8 |
| Cheddar & herbs rice dish | 1 cup | 310 | 48 | 3 | 45 | 10 | 7 |
| Chicken & vegetable rice | 1 cup | 290 | 51 | 3 | 48 | 8 | 3 |
| Chicken vermicelli rice dish | 1 cup | 290 | 52 | 3 | 49 | 9 | 3 |
| Herb & butter rice dish | 1 cup | 280 | 53 | 3 | 50 | 8 | 4 |
| Mexican style rice | 1 cup | 265 | 45 | 3 | 42 | 7 | 4 |
| Rice pilaf | 1 cup | 305 | 54 | 3 | 51 | 8 | 4 |
| Spanish rice dish | 1 cup | 270 | 45 | 3 | 42 | 7 | 4 |
| **Rice Cake**, plain | 1 | 35 | 7 | Tr | 7 | 1 | Tr |

| | Serving Size | Calories (g) | Total Carbs(g) | Fiber (g) | Net Carbs(g) | Protein (g) | Fat (g) |
|---|---|---|---|---|---|---|---|
| Butter flavor | 1 | 40 | 8 | Tr | 8 | 1 | Tr |
| Carmel | 1 | 48 | 11 | Tr | 11 | 1 | Tr |
| *Rice Krispies Treat* | 1 bar | 90 | 18 | Tr | 18 | 1 | 2 |
| **Rigatoni,** meat sauce *Lean Cuisine entrée* | 1 meal | 260 | 25 | 2 | 23 | 18 | 10 |
| **Roast Beef** – see Beef | ... | ... | . | . | . | . | . |
| **Roast Beef Sandwich** 3 oz meat w/ sauce | 1 avg | 390 | 33 | 3 | 30 | 23 | 19 |
| **Rolls** – see Bread | ... | ... | . | . | . | . | . |
| *Rosemary, dried spice* | *1/2 tsp* | *2* | *Tr* | *Tr* | *Tr* | *Tr* | *0* |
| **Rutabaga,** cubed, cooked | 1 cup | 65 | 15 | 3 | 12 | 2 | Tr |
| *Saccharin sweetener* | *1 pkt* | *0* | *Tr* | *0* | *Tr* | *0* | *0* |
| *Sage, dried spice* | *½ tsp* | *1* | *Tr* | *Tr* | *Tr* | *Tr* | *0* |
| SALAD DRESSING | | | | | | | |
| *Blue cheese, regular* | *1 Tbsp* | *75* | *1* | *0* | *1* | *1* | *8* |
| *Blue cheese, low calorie* | *1 Tbsp* | *15* | *1* | *0* | *1* | *1* | *1* |
| *Buttermilk, regular* | *1 Tbsp* | *60* | *1* | *0* | *1* | *Tr* | *6* |
| *Buttermilk, low calorie* | *1 Tbsp* | *15* | *1* | *0* | *1* | *Tr* | *1* |
| *Caesar, regular* | *1 Tbsp* | *80* | *Tr* | *Tr* | *Tr* | *Tr* | *8* |
| *Caesar, low calorie* | *1 Tbsp* | *17* | *3* | *Tr* | *3* | *Tr* | *1* |
| *French, regular* | *1 Tbsp* | *70* | *3* | *0* | *3* | *Tr* | *6* |
| *French, low calorie* | *1 Tbsp* | *25* | *4* | *0* | *4* | *Tr* | *1* |
| *Honey Dijon, regular* | *1 Tbsp* | *70* | *3* | *0* | *3* | *Tr* | *6* |
| *Honey Dijon, fat free* | *1 Tbsp* | *25* | *4* | *0* | *4* | *Tr* | *1* |
| *Italian, regular* | *1 Tbsp* | *70* | *1* | *0* | *1* | *Tr* | *7* |
| *Italian, low calorie* | *1 Tbsp* | *16* | *1* | *0* | *1* | *Tr* | *1* |
| *Mayonnaise, regular* | *1 Tbsp* | *100* | *Tr* | *0* | *Tr* | *Tr* | *11* |
| *Mayonnaise, light* | *1 Tbsp* | *50* | *1* | *0* | *1* | *Tr* | *5* |
| *Mayonnaise, fat free* | *1 Tbsp* | *10* | *2* | *0* | *2* | *Tr* | *0* |
| *Ranch, regular* | *1 Tbsp* | *70* | *2* | *0* | *2* | *Tr* | *6* |
| *Ranch, low calorie* | *1 Tbsp* | *20* | *3* | *0* | *3* | *Tr* | *1* |
| *Russian, regular* | *1 Tbsp* | *75* | *2* | *0* | *2* | *Tr* | *8* |
| *Russian, low calorie* | *1 Tbsp* | *25* | *4* | *Tr* | *4* | *Tr* | *1* |
| *Thousand Island, regular* | *1 Tbsp* | *65* | *2* | *0* | *2* | *Tr* | *6* |
| *Thousand Island, low calorie* | *1 Tbsp* | *26* | *2* | *Tr* | *2* | *Tr* | *2* |

| | Serving Size | Calories (g) | Total Carbs(g) | Fiber (g) | Net Carbs(g) | Protein (g) | Fat (g) |
|---|---|---|---|---|---|---|---|
| **Zero Carb Salad Dressing** | | | | | | | |
| *Nature's Flavors* | | | | | | | |
| **Carbfree Blue Cheese** | **2 Tbsp** | **30** | **0** | **0** | **0** | **1** | **3** |
| **Carbfree French** | **2 Tbsp** | **30** | **0** | **0** | **0** | **1** | **3** |
| **Salad, Tossed** | | | | | | | |
| All Vegetable salad, no dressing | 1½ cups | 60 | 11 | 4 | 7 | 3 | Tr |
| Salad w/egg & cheese | | | | | | | |
| **no dressing** | **1½ cups** | **120** | **5** | **1** | **4** | **9** | **7** |
| w/regular dressing, any type | 1½ cups | 200 | 6 | 1 | 5 | 10 | 17 |
| w/light dressing, any type | 1½ cups | 135 | 9 | 1 | 8 | 9 | 7 |
| Salad w/grilled chicken or turkey | | | | | | | |
| no dressing | 1½ cups | 150 | 11 | 1 | 10 | 19 | 3 |
| w/regular dressing, any type | 1½ cups | 250 | 12 | 1 | 11 | 20 | 13 |
| w/light dressing, any type | 1½ cups | 175 | 15 | 1 | 14 | 19 | 3 |
| (Also see Pasta Salad, Potato Salad, & other specific listings) | | | | | | | |
| **Salami** | | | | | | | |
| **Regular, any meat** | **2 oz** | **130** | **1** | **0** | **1** | **7** | **11** |
| **Lowfat, Turkey or Chicken, thin 1/8" slices** | **2 slices** | **80** | **1** | **0** | **1** | **8** | **5** |
| **Cotto** | **2 slices** | **95** | **1** | **0** | **1** | **7** | **7** |
| **Dried type, 3" x ⅛" slices** | **2 slices** | **95** | **1** | **0** | **1** | **6** | **7** |
| **Hard** | **1 oz** | **110** | **1** | **0** | **1** | **6** | **9** |
| Salisbury Steak | | | | | | | |
| *Banquet entrée* | 1 meal | 220 | 8 | 1 | 7 | 9 | 16 |
| *Morton's entrée* | 1 meal | 210 | 23 | 2 | 21 | 9 | 9 |
| *Stouffer's entrée* | 1 meal | 240 | 10 | 1 | 9 | 17 | 15 |
| *Weight Watchers entrée* | 1 meal | 150 | 24 | 1 | 23 | 19 | 9 |
| **Salsa** | **1 Tbsp** | **4** | **1** | **Tr** | **Tr** | **Tr** | **Tr** |

| | Serving Size | Calories (g) | Total Carbs (g) | Fiber (g) | Net Carbs (g) | Protein (g) | Fat (g) |
|---|---|---|---|---|---|---|---|
| **Salt** | | | | | | | |
| *Regular* | ½ tsp | 0 | 0 | 0 | 0 | 0 | 0 |
| *Reduced sodium* | ½ tsp | 0 | 0 | 0 | 0 | 0 | 0 |
| *Seasoned* | ½ tsp | 5 | Tr | Tr | Tr | Tr | Tr |
| Sandwich, w/ 2.5 oz Meat on Lg 6" bun, sub, or kaiser roll | | | | | | | |
| Cold Cuts, mixed meats w/ sauce, cheese, tomato, lettuce | 1 | 455 | 51 | 2 | 49 | 22 | 19 |
| Ham & Cheese w/ sauce | 1 | 550 | 57 | 4 | 53 | 33 | 21 |
| Roast Beef w/ mayo, tomato, lettuce | 1 | 410 | 44 | 2 | 42 | 29 | 13 |
| Tuna salad w/ mayo, lettuce | 1 | 585 | 55 | 2 | 53 | 30 | 28 |
| Sandwich Meat – see Lunch Meat | ... | ... | . | . | . | . | . |
| **Sandwich Spread** | 1 Tbsp | 35 | 2 | Tr | 2 | 1 | 3 |
| **SAUCE** | | | | | | | |
| *A1 Steak Sauce* | 1 Tbsp | 15 | 3 | Tr | 3 | 0 | 0 |
| *Barbecue sauce, regular* | 1 Tbsp | 20 | 4 | 1 | 3 | Tr | Tr |
| Barbecue, thick or honey | 1 Tbsp | 40 | 8 | Tr | 8 | Tr | 1 |
| *Catsup* | 1 Tbsp | 18 | 4 | Tr | 4 | Tr | Tr |
| *Cheese sauce* | ¼ cup | 110 | 4 | Tr | 4 | 4 | 8 |
| Chili sauce | ¼ cup | 60 | 13 | 3 | 10 | 1 | Tr |
| *Duck Sauce* | 1 Tbsp | 20 | 4 | Tr | 4 | 0 | 0 |
| Hoison sauce | 1 Tbsp | 35 | 7 | Tr | 6 | 1 | 1 |
| *Hollandaise sauce* | 1 Tbsp | 18 | 2 | Tr | 2 | 1 | 1 |
| *Horseradish, prepared* | 1 tsp | 4 | 1 | Tr | 1 | Tr | Tr |
| *Hot sauce* | 1 tsp | 1 | Tr | Tr | Tr | Tr | Tr |
| *Marinara sauce* | ¼ cup | 36 | 5 | 1 | 4 | 1 | 1 |
| *Mayonnaise, regular* | 1 Tbsp | 100 | Tr | 0 | Tr | Tr | 11 |
| *Mayonnaise, light* | 1 Tbsp | 50 | 1 | 0 | 1 | Tr | 5 |
| *Mayonnaise, fat free* | 1 Tbsp | 10 | 2 | 0 | 2 | Tr | 0 |
| *Mustard, regular* | 1 tsp | 4 | Tr | Tr | Tr | Tr | Tr |
| *Mustard, hot or honey* | 1 tsp | 8 | 2 | Tr | 2 | Tr | Tr |
| *Oyster sauce* | 1 Tbsp | 5 | 1 | Tr | Tr | Tr | Tr |
| *Pasta sauce* | ¼ cup | 35 | 5 | 1 | 4 | 1 | 1 |

| | Serving Size | Calories (g) | Total Carbs(g) | Fiber (g) | Net Carbs(g) | Protein (g) | Fat (g) |
|---|---|---|---|---|---|---|---|
| *Pepper sauce, hot* | *1 tsp* | *1* | *Tr* | *Tr* | *Tr* | *Tr* | *Tr* |
| Pickle Relish | 1 Tbsp | 20 | 5 | Tr | 5 | Tr | Tr |
| *Pizza sauce* | *¼ cup* | *35* | *5* | *1* | *4* | *1* | *1* |
| *Salsa* | *1 Tbsp* | *4* | *1* | *Tr* | *Tr* | *Tr* | *Tr* |
| *Sloppy Joe sauce* | | | | | | | |
| *w/meat* | *1 Tbsp* | *45* | *5* | *1* | *4* | *2* | *2* |
| *Soy sauce* | *1 Tbsp* | *10* | *1* | *Tr* | *Tr* | *1* | *Tr* |
| *Spaghetti sauce* | *¼ cup* | *36* | *5* | *1* | *4* | *1* | *1* |
| *Steak sauce* | *1 Tbsp* | *15* | *3* | *Tr* | *3* | *0* | *0* |
| *Sweet & Sour sauce* | *1 Tbsp* | *20* | *4* | *Tr* | *4* | *0* | *0* |
| *Szechuan sauce* | *1 Tbsp* | *20* | *3* | *Tr* | *3* | *1* | *Tr* |
| *Tabasco sauce* | *1 tsp* | *1* | *Tr* | *Tr* | *Tr* | *Tr* | *Tr* |
| *Taco sauce* | *1 Tbsp* | *10* | *2* | *Tr* | *2* | *Tr* | *Tr* |
| *Tamari sauce* | *1 Tbsp* | *11* | *1* | *0* | *1* | *2* | *0* |
| *Tartar sauce* | *1 Tbsp* | *45* | *2* | *Tr* | *2* | *0* | *4* |
| *Teriyaki sauce* | *1 Tbsp* | *20* | *4* | *Tr* | *4* | *1* | *Tr* |
| Tomato sauce | ½ cup | 37 | 9 | 2 | 7 | 1 | Tr |
| White sauce | ¼ cup | 92 | 6 | Tr | 6 | 3 | 6 |
| *Worcestershire sauce* | *1 Tbsp* | *12* | *3* | *Tr* | *3* | *0* | *0* |
| Zero Carb Sauce | | | | | | | |
| *Nature's Flavors* | | | | | | | |
| **Barbecue sauce** | 2 Tbsp | 0 | 0 | 0 | 0 | 0 | 0 |
| **Honey Mustard** | | | | | | | |
| **sauce** | 2 Tbsp | 0 | 0 | 0 | 0 | 0 | 0 |
| *Sauerkraut* | *1 cup* | *45* | *10* | *6* | *4* | *2* | *Tr* |
| Sausage | | | | | | | |
| *Breakfast link, small* | *1 link* | *70* | *Tr* | *0* | *Tr* | *3* | *6* |
| *Breakfast patty, small* | *1 patty* | *80* | *Tr* | *0* | *Tr* | *3* | *7* |
| *Beef or Pork sausage* | *2 oz* | *120* | *1* | *0* | *1* | *7* | *10* |
| *Chicken or Turkey* | | | | | | | |
| *sausage* | *2 oz* | *98* | *1* | *0* | *1* | *6* | *8* |
| Lowfat sausage, beef or pork | 2 oz | 80 | 6 | 0 | 6 | 7 | 2 |
| Lowfat sausage,chicken or turkey | 2 oz | 78 | 6 | 0 | 6 | 7 | 2 |
| Fat free sausage, beef or pork | 2 oz | 60 | 6 | 0 | 6 | 7 | 0 |
| Fat free sausage, chicken or turkey | 2 oz | 58 | 6 | 0 | 6 | 7 | 0 |
| *Polish sausage, Kielbasa* | *2 oz* | *120* | *Tr* | *0* | *Tr* | *8* | *10* |

| | Serving Size | Calories (g) | Total Carbs(g) | Fiber (g) | Net Carbs(g) | Protein (g) | Fat (g) |
|---|---|---|---|---|---|---|---|
| *Vienna sausage, 2" links* | *2 links* | *90* | *Tr* | *0* | *Tr* | *4* | *8* |
| Scallop – see Fish/Seafood | ... | ... | . | . | . | . | . |
| Seafood – see Fish/Seafood | ... | ... | . | . | . | . | . |
| Seasoning – see specific listings | ... | ... | . | . | . | . | . |
| *Blended Seasoning w/ salt, garlic, onion, paprika, papain* | *½ tsp* | *2* | *Tr* | *Tr* | *Tr* | *Tr* | *0* |
| Seaweed | | | | | | | |
| *Kelp, raw* | *2 Tbsp* | *4* | *1* | *Tr* | *Tr* | *Tr* | *Tr* |
| *Spirulina, dried* | *1 Tbsp* | *3* | *Tr* | *Tr* | *Tr* | *1* | *Tr* |
| *Thin wrap sheets* | *1 sheet* | *10* | *2* | *Tr* | *2* | *1* | *Tr* |
| Seeds | | | | | | | |
| *Pumpkin seeds, roasted* | *1 oz* | *148* | *4* | *1* | *3* | *9* | *12* |
| *Sesame seeds, plain* | *1 Tbsp* | *47* | *1* | *Tr* | *Tr* | *2* | *4* |
| *Sesame seeds, butter, roasted* | *1 Tbsp* | *90* | *3* | *1* | *2* | *3* | *8* |
| *Soybean seeds, dried, boiled* | *½ cup* | *145* | *9* | *5* | *4* | *15* | *7* |
| *Sunflower seeds, dry roasted* | *1 oz* | *165* | *7* | *3* | *4* | *5* | *14* |
| (Also see specific listings) | | | | | | | |
| *Shallot, raw, chopped* | *1 Tbsp* | *7* | *2* | *Tr* | *2* | *Tr* | *Tr* |
| Shark – see Fish | ... | ... | . | . | . | . | . |
| Sherbet, Orange | ½ cup | 100 | 22 | 0 | 22 | 1 | 1 |
| Rainbow | ½ cup | 105 | 23 | 0 | 23 | 1 | 1 |
| *Shortening, regular cottonseed & soybean blend* | *1 cup* | *1810* | *0* | *0* | *0* | *0* | *205* |
| | *1 Tbsp* | *115* | *0* | *0* | *0* | *0* | *13* |
| Shrimp – see Fish/Seafood & specific entrées | ... | ... | . | . | . | . | . |

| | Serving Size | Calories (g) | Total Carbs(g) | Fiber (g) | Net Carbs(g) | Protein (g) | Fat (g) |
|---|---|---|---|---|---|---|---|
| **Shrimp & Broccoli** | | | | | | | |
| w/creamy white sauce | 1 cup | 270 | 29 | 1 | 28 | 15 | 10 |
| **Shrimp & Pasta** | | | | | | | |
| w/creamy white sauce | 1 cup | 300 | 34 | 1 | 33 | 14 | 13 |
| **Shrimp & Vegetables** | | | | | | | |
| Hunan style | 1 cup | 240 | 30 | 3 | 27 | 14 | 7 |
| **Shrimp & Vegetables** | | | | | | | |
| w/szechuan sauce | 1 cup | 230 | 30 | 3 | 27 | 14 | 6 |
| **Shrimp Marinara** | | | | | | | |
| *Weight Watchers entrée* | 1 meal | 200 | 37 | 1 | 36 | 8 | 2 |
| **Sirloin Steak** – see Beef | ... | ... | . | . | . | . | . |
| **Snack Mix,** *Chex Mix* | ¾ cup | 120 | 18 | 2 | 16 | 3 | 5 |
| **Sorbet,** orange or raspberry | ½ cup | 120 | 30 | 0 | 30 | 0 | 0 |
| ***Soufflé, regular type*** | *1 cup* | *250* | *3* | *1* | *2* | *12* | *20* |
| **SOUP** *(as prep)* | | | | | | | |
| ***Bouillon cube, regular,*** | | | | | | | |
| ***all varieties,*** | | | | | | | |
| ***makes 1 cup*** | *1 cube* | *5* | *1* | *Tr* | *Tr* | *Tr* | *Tr* |
| ***Bouillon packet, low*** | | | | | | | |
| ***sodium, all varieties,*** | | | | | | | |
| ***makes 1 cup*** | *1 pkt* | *15* | *3* | *Tr* | *3* | *Tr* | *Tr* |
| ***Broth, consommé,*** | | | | | | | |
| ***all varieties*** | *1 cup* | *20* | *3* | *Tr* | *3* | *1* | *Tr* |
| Bean w/ Ham soup | 1 cup | 185 | 24 | 9 | 15 | 8 | 7 |
| Bean w/ Pork soup | 1 cup | 175 | 23 | 9 | 14 | 8 | 6 |
| Beef Noodle soup | 1 cup | 83 | 9 | 1 | 8 | 5 | 3 |
| Chicken Noodle soup, regular | 1 cup | 75 | 9 | 1 | 8 | 4 | 2 |
| Chicken Noodle soup, chunky | 1 cup | 175 | 17 | 4 | 13 | 13 | 6 |
| Chicken & Rice soup | 1 cup | 70 | 8 | 1 | 7 | 5 | 2 |
| Chicken & Vegetable, regular | 1 cup | 90 | 12 | 1 | 11 | 6 | 1 |
| Chicken & Vegetable, chunky | 1 cup | 165 | 19 | 1 | 18 | 12 | 5 |
| Clam Chowder, Manhattan | 1 cup | 85 | 12 | 2 | 10 | 2 | 2 |
| Clam Chowder, New England | 1 cup | 165 | 17 | 2 | 15 | 9 | 7 |

| | Serving Size | Calories (g) | Total Carbs(g) | Fiber (g) | Net Carbs(g) | Protein (g) | Fat (g) |
|---|---|---|---|---|---|---|---|
| Clam Chowder, Low fat, New England | 1 cup | 115 | 20 | 1 | 19 | 5 | 2 |
| Cream of Broccoli soup | | | | | | | |
| prep w/ water | 1 cup | 125 | 8 | 1 | 7 | 2 | 9 |
| prep w/ milk | 1 cup | 195 | 14 | 1 | 13 | 6 | 14 |
| Cream of Chicken soup | | | | | | | |
| prep w/ water | 1 cup | 117 | 9 | Tr | 9 | 3 | 7 |
| prep w/ milk | 1 cup | 190 | 15 | Tr | 15 | 7 | 11 |
| Cream of Mushroom soup | | | | | | | |
| prep w/ water | 1 cup | 130 | 9 | 1 | 8 | 2 | 9 |
| prep w/ milk | 1 cup | 200 | 15 | 1 | 14 | 6 | 14 |
| Lentil soup, low fat | 1 cup | 125 | 20 | 6 | 14 | 8 | 2 |
| Minestrone | 1 cup | 85 | 11 | 1 | 10 | 4 | 3 |
| Onion soup | 1 cup | 100 | 19 | 4 | 15 | 4 | 2 |
| Pea soup | 1 cup | 160 | 26 | 3 | 23 | 9 | 3 |
| Potato w/ bean soup | 1 cup | 170 | 23 | 2 | 21 | 6 | 7 |
| Ramen Beef Noodle soup | 1 cup | 190 | 26 | 1 | 25 | 4 | 8 |
| Ramen Chicken Noodle soup | 1 cup | 190 | 26 | 1 | 25 | 4 | 8 |
| Ramen Mushroom Noodle soup | 1 cup | 180 | 26 | 1 | 25 | 4 | 7 |
| Tomato soup, prep w/ water | 1 cup | 85 | 17 | 1 | 16 | 2 | 2 |
| Tomato soup, prep w/ milk | 1 cup | 160 | 22 | 1 | 21 | 6 | 6 |
| Vegetable soup | 1 cup | 72 | 12 | 1 | 11 | 2 | 2 |
| Vegetable Beef soup | 1 cup | 90 | 11 | 1 | 10 | 7 | 2 |
| Wisconsin Cheese soup | 1 cup | 280 | 20 | 2 | 18 | 10 | 18 |
| **Sour cream** | | | | | | | |
| Regular | 1 cup | 495 | 10 | 0 | 10 | 7 | 48 |
| ***Regular*** | ***1 Tbsp*** | ***25*** | ***1*** | ***0*** | ***1*** | ***Tr*** | ***3*** |
| ***Reduced fat*** | ***1 Tbsp*** | ***20*** | ***1*** | ***0*** | ***1*** | ***Tr*** | ***2*** |
| ***Fat free*** | ***1 Tbsp*** | ***12*** | ***2*** | ***0*** | ***2*** | ***Tr*** | ***0*** |
| **Soy Burger**, broiled | 1 patty | 100 | 9 | 3 | 6 | 15 | 1 |
| **Soybeans** | | | | | | | |
| ***dried mature seeds, cooked*** | ***½ cup*** | ***145*** | ***9*** | ***5*** | ***4*** | ***15*** | ***7*** |
| **Spaghetti** | | | | | | | |
| Plain, cooked | 1 cup | 195 | 40 | 2 | 38 | 7 | 1 |

| | Serving Size | Calories (g) | Total Carbs(g) | Fiber (g) | Net Carbs(g) | Protein (g) | Fat (g) |
|---|---|---|---|---|---|---|---|
| With cheese & tomato sauce | 1 cup | 220 | 41 | 3 | 38 | 8 | 2 |
| With meatballs in tomato sauce | 1 cup | 240 | 41 | 3 | 38 | 7 | 4 |
| With tomato sauce | 1 cup | 260 | 31 | 3 | 28 | 11 | 10 |
| **Spaghetti Bolognese, w/ meat sauce,** *Healthy Choice* **entrée** | 1 meal | 255 | 43 | 5 | 38 | 14 | 3 |
| **Spare Ribs** – see Pork | ... | ... | . | . | | . | . |
| **Spice** – see specific listings | | | | | | | |
| **Blended Spice w/ basil, garlic, oregano, rosemary, thyme** | **½ tsp** | **3** | **Tr** | **Tr** | **Tr** | **Tr** | **0** |
| **Spinach** | | | | | | | |
| **Fresh, raw, chopped** | **1 cup** | **7** | **1** | **Tr** | **Tr** | **1** | **Tr** |
| **Fresh, chopped, cooked** | **1 cup** | **41** | **7** | **4** | **3** | **5** | **Tr** |
| **Frozen, chopped, cooked** | **1 cup** | **53** | **10** | **6** | **4** | **6** | **Tr** |
| **Canned, cooked** | **1 cup** | **50** | **7** | **5** | **2** | **6** | **Tr** |
| **Spinach Soufflé** | **1 cup** | **220** | **3** | **1** | **2** | **11** | **18** |
| Spread | | | | | | | |
| **Cheese Spread** | **1 Tbsp** | **40** | **1** | **0** | **1** | **3** | **3** |
| **Sandwich Spread** | **1 Tbsp** | **35** | **2** | **Tr** | **2** | **1** | **3** |
| (also see spreads in Margarine) | | | | | | | |
| Squash | | | | | | | |
| Butternut squash | ¾ cup | 150 | 25 | 4 | 21 | 2 | 6 |
| **Summer, raw, sliced** | **1 cup** | **23** | **5** | **2** | **3** | **1** | **Tr** |
| Summer, cooked, slices | 1 cup | 36 | 8 | 3 | 5 | 2 | 1 |
| Winter, baked, cubes | 1 cup | 80 | 18 | 6 | 12 | 2 | 1 |
| Winter, frozen, cooked, mashed | 1 cup | 94 | 24 | 2 | 22 | 3 | Tr |
| **Squash Casserole** | ¾ cup | 330 | 20 | 6 | 14 | 7 | 24 |
| **Steak** – see Beef | ... | ... | . | . | | . | . |
| **Steak Sauce, A1** | **1 Tbsp** | **15** | **3** | **Tr** | **3** | **0** | **0** |

| | Serving Size | Calories (g) | Total Carbs(g) | Fiber (g) | Net Carbs(g) | Protein (g) | Fat (g) |
|---|---|---|---|---|---|---|---|
| **Strawberries** | | | | | | | |
| Fresh, med size, 1 ¼" dia | 10 | 40 | 9 | 3 | 6 | 1 | Tr |
| Fresh, sliced | 1 cup | 50 | 12 | 4 | 8 | 1 | 1 |
| Frozen, sweetened, | | | | | | | |
| thawed | 1 cup | 245 | 66 | 5 | 61 | 1 | Tr |
| **Strawberry Shortcake** | 1 avg | 275 | 20 | 2 | 18 | 6 | 15 |
| **Streusel** (avg size slice) | | | | | | | |
| Apple | 1 slice | 240 | 33 | 2 | 31 | 4 | 17 |
| Cherry | 1 slice | 205 | 30 | 2 | 28 | 4 | 16 |
| **Stuffing,** as prep | | | | | | | |
| Traditional stuffing, | | | | | | | |
| seasoned, meat flavored | 1 cup | 360 | 44 | 6 | 38 | 6 | 18 |
| Corn bread stuffing, | | | | | | | |
| seasoned | 1 cup | 345 | 42 | 5 | 37 | 5 | 17 |
| **Succotash** | ½ cup | 80 | 17 | 3 | 14 | 3 | 1 |
| **Sugar** | | | | | | | |
| *White, regular, granulated* | | | | | | | |
| One cup | 1 cup | 774 | 200 | 0 | 200 | 0 | 0 |
| One tablespoon | 1 Tbsp | 45 | 12 | 0 | 12 | 0 | 0 |
| ***One teaspoon*** | *1 tsp* | *15* | *4* | *0* | *4* | *0* | *0* |
| Restaurant size packet | 1 pkt | 24 | 6 | 0 | 6 | 0 | 0 |
| *White, Confectioner's,* | | | | | | | |
| *Powdered* | | | | | | | |
| Unsifted, one cup | 1 cup | 31 | 8 | 0 | 8 | 0 | 0 |
| Unsifted | 1 Tbsp | 467 | 119 | 0 | 119 | 0 | 0 |
| *Brown Sugar* | | | | | | | |
| Packed, one cup | 1 cup | 827 | 214 | 0 | 214 | 0 | 0 |
| Not packed, one cup | 1 cup | 545 | 141 | 0 | 141 | 0 | 0 |
| Not packed, | | | | | | | |
| one tablespoon | 1 Tbsp | 34 | 9 | 0 | 9 | 0 | 0 |
| **Sugar Substitute** | | | | | | | |
| ***Aspartame*** | | | | | | | |
| ***sweetener*** | *1 pkt* | *0* | *Tr* | *0* | *Tr* | *0* | *0* |
| ***Saccharine*** | | | | | | | |
| ***sweetener*** | *1 pkt* | *0* | *Tr* | *0* | *Tr* | *0* | *0* |
| **Sundae** (small serving) | | | | | | | |
| Hot Fudge | 1 | 285 | 48 | 1 | 47 | 6 | 9 |
| Strawberry | 1 | 230 | 45 | 1 | 44 | 6 | 3 |
| Strawberry Yogurt | 1 | 275 | 59 | 1 | 58 | 9 | 1 |

|  | Serving Size | Calories (g) | Total Carbs(g) | Fiber (g) | Net Carbs(g) | Protein (g) | Fat (g) |
|---|---|---|---|---|---|---|---|
| **Swedish Meatballs** | | | | | | | |
| *Celentano,* | | | | | | | |
| 6 meatball meal | 1 meal | 260 | 5 | Tr | 5 | 12 | 19 |
| *Lean Cuisine entrée* | 1 meal | 290 | 35 | 1 | 34 | 22 | 7 |
| *Weight Watchers entrée* | 1 meal | 290 | 34 | 1 | 33 | 18 | 7 |
| ***Sweet 'N Low*** | *1 pkt* | *0* | *Tr* | *0* | *Tr* | *0* | *0* |
| **Sweet Potato** | | | | | | | |
| Baked w/skin 4" x 2" | 1 whole | 165 | 38 | 4 | 34 | 3 | Tr |
| Baked or Boiled | | | | | | | |
| w/o skin 4" x 2" | 1 whole | 150 | 35 | 3 | 32 | 3 | Tr |
| Boiled, peeled, mashed | ½ cup | 170 | 30 | 3 | 27 | 3 | 3 |
| Candied, 2 ½" x 2" pieces | 1 piece | 145 | 29 | 3 | 26 | 1 | 3 |
| Canned in syrup, drained | 1 cup | 210 | 50 | 6 | 44 | 3 | 1 |
| Canned, vacuum pack, | | | | | | | |
| mashed | 1 cup | 230 | 54 | 5 | 49 | 4 | 1 |
| Whipped, frozen, heated | ½ cup | 140 | 18 | 3 | 15 | 2 | 6 |
| **Sweet Potato Casserole** | ¾ cup | 280 | 39 | 4 | 35 | 3 | 18 |
| **Sweet Roll** | ... | ... | . | . | . | . | . |
| – see specific listings | | | | | | | |
| **Syrup** | | | | | | | |
| Butterscotch | 1 Tbsp | 60 | 12 | Tr | 12 | 0 | 1 |
| Chocolate, thin | 1 Tbsp | 55 | 12 | Tr | 12 | Tr | Tr |
| Chocolate fudge, thick | 1 Tbsp | 65 | 12 | 1 | 11 | 1 | 2 |
| Corn, light | 1 Tbsp | 56 | 15 | 0 | 15 | 0 | 0 |
| Maple | 1 Tbsp | 52 | 13 | 0 | 13 | 0 | Tr |
| Molasses, blackstrap | 1 Tbsp | 47 | 12 | 0 | 12 | 0 | 0 |
| | 1 cup | 771 | 199 | 0 | 199 | 0 | 0 |
| **Pancake Syrup/Table** | | | | | | | |
| **Syrup** | | | | | | | |
| Regular | 1 Tbsp | 55 | 14 | 0 | 14 | 0 | 0 |
| Light, reduced calorie | 1 Tbsp | 25 | 7 | 0 | 7 | 0 | 0 |
| ***Sugar free*** | *1 Tbsp* | *8* | *3* | *Tr* | *3* | *0* | *0* |
| *Zero Carb Syrup* | | | | | | | |
| *Nature's Flavors* | | | | | | | |
| ***Apple*** | *2 Tbsp* | *0* | *0* | *0* | *0* | *0* | *0* |
| ***Brown Sugar*** | *2 Tbsp* | *0* | *0* | *0* | *0* | *0* | *0* |
| ***Chocolate*** | *2 Tbsp* | *0* | *0* | *0* | *0* | *0* | *0* |
| ***Maple*** | *1 Tbsp* | *0* | *0* | *0* | *0* | *0* | *0* |

| | Serving Size | Calories (g) | Total Carbs(g) | Fiber (g) | Net Carbs(g) | Protein (g) | Fat (g) |
|---|---|---|---|---|---|---|---|
| **Taco** (w/hard or soft shell) | | | | | | | |
| Regular size, with beef | 1 | 210 | 18 | 2 | 16 | 11 | 11 |
| Regular size, with chicken | 1 | 190 | 17 | 2 | 15 | 13 | 8 |
| Large, with steak or beef | 1 | 280 | 20 | 2 | 18 | 13 | 17 |
| X-Lg, double decker, with beef | 1 | 365 | 27 | 2 | 25 | 21 | 18 |
| **Taco Salad** w/ ground beef, cheese, taco shell | 1 | 275 | 24 | 2 | 22 | 13 | 15 |
| **Taco Shell** (shell only) | | | | | | | |
| Thin shell, 6" dia | 1 | 60 | 8 | 1 | 7 | 1 | 3 |
| Large shell | 1 | 100 | 13 | 1 | 12 | 2 | 5 |
| ***Tahini, from toasted kernels*** | ***1 Tbsp*** | ***90*** | ***3*** | ***1*** | ***2*** | ***3*** | ***8*** |
| **Tamale**, meatless | 2 pieces | 215 | 30 | 1 | 29 | 6 | 8 |
| *Beef, Swanson entrée* | 1 meal | 350 | 46 | 1 | 45 | 13 | 13 |
| *Chicken, Swanson entrée* | 1 meal | 325 | 45 | 1 | 44 | 8 | 12 |
| **Tangerine,** fresh, med, 2 ½" dia | 1 | 37 | 9 | 2 | 7 | 1 | Tr |
| **Tapioca,** pearl, dry | 1 cup | 545 | 135 | 1 | 134 | Tr | Tr |
| ***Taro Leaf, steamed*** | ***1/2 cup*** | ***18*** | ***4*** | ***2*** | ***2*** | ***1*** | ***Tr*** |
| ***Tarragon, ground*** | ***1 tsp*** | ***5*** | ***1*** | ***Tr*** | ***Tr*** | ***Tr*** | ***Tr*** |
| **Tater Tots** fried potatoes | 10 | 175 | 24 | 3 | 21 | 3 | 8 |
| **T-bone Steak** – see Beef | ... | ... | . | . | . | . | . |
| **Teriyaki** – see Beef Teriyaki or Chicken Teriyaki | ... | ... | . | . | . | . | . |
| ***Thyme, dried spice*** | ***1/2 tsp*** | ***2*** | ***Tr*** | ***Tr*** | ***Tr*** | ***Tr*** | ***0*** |
| **Toaster Pastry** (Pop Tart) | | | | | | | |
| Apple, frosted | 1 pastry | 200 | 37 | 1 | 36 | 2 | 5 |
| Apple, unfrosted | 1 pastry | 185 | 34 | 1 | 33 | 2 | 5 |
| Blueberry, frosted | 1 pastry | 200 | 37 | 1 | 36 | 2 | 5 |
| Blueberry, unfrosted | 1 pastry | 185 | 34 | 1 | 33 | 2 | 5 |
| Brown sugar, cinnamon, frosted | 1 pastry | 190 | 36 | 1 | 35 | 2 | 5 |
| Chocolate, frosted | 1 pastry | 200 | 37 | 1 | 36 | 3 | 5 |
| Chocolate fudge, frosted | 1 pastry | 200 | 36 | 1 | 35 | 3 | 5 |
| Grape, frosted | 1 pastry | 200 | 37 | 1 | 36 | 2 | 5 |
| Grape, unfrosted | 1 pastry | 185 | 34 | 1 | 33 | 2 | 5 |

| | Serving Size | Calories (g) | Total Carbs(g) | Fiber (g) | Net Carbs(g) | Protein (g) | Fat (g) |
|---|---|---|---|---|---|---|---|
| Lowfat, frosted, any variety | 1 pastry | 170 | 37 | 1 | 36 | 2 | 2 |
| Lowfat, unfrosted, any variety | 1 pastry | 155 | 33 | 1 | 32 | 2 | 2 |
| S'mores, frosted | 1 pastry | 220 | 39 | 1 | 38 | 2 | 6 |
| Strawberry, frosted | 1 pastry | 200 | 37 | 1 | 36 | 2 | 5 |
| Strawberry, unfrosted | 1 pastry | 185 | 34 | 1 | 33 | 2 | 5 |
| *Tofu, plain, cooked, 4 oz* | *½ cup* | *80* | *2* | *Tr* | *2* | *9* | *4* |
| Tomatillos, *raw, medium size* | *2* | *22* | *4* | *1* | *3* | *Tr* | *Tr* |
| Tomato | | | | | | | |
| Fresh, raw, 2 ½" dia | 1 whole | 26 | 6 | 1 | 5 | 1 | Tr |
| *Cherry tomato fresh, raw* | *1 whole* | *4* | *1* | *Tr* | *Tr* | *Tr* | *Tr* |
| *Fresh, slices, ¼" thick* | *1 slice* | *4* | *1* | *Tr* | *Tr* | *Tr* | *Tr* |
| Fresh, chopped or sliced | 1 cup | 38 | 8 | 2 | 6 | 2 | 1 |
| Canned, liquids and solids | 1 cup | 46 | 10 | 2 | 8 | 2 | Tr |
| Stewed, fresh or canned | 1 cup | 70 | 17 | 3 | 14 | 2 | 1 |
| Sun Dried | | | | | | | |
| *Plain* | *1 piece* | *5* | *1* | *Tr* | *Tr* | *Tr* | *Tr* |
| *Packed in oil, drained* | *1 piece* | *6* | *1* | *Tr* | *Tr* | *Tr* | *Tr* |
| Tomato Paste | 1 cup | 215 | 51 | 11 | 40 | 10 | 1 |
| Tomato Puree | 1 cup | 100 | 24 | 5 | 19 | 4 | Tr |
| Tomato Sauce | 1 cup | 74 | 18 | 3 | 15 | 3 | Tr |
| Topping, for dessert | | | | | | | |
| Butterscotch, regular | 1 Tbsp | 60 | 12 | Tr | 12 | 0 | 1 |
| Butterscotch, light | 1 Tbsp | 30 | 8 | Tr | 8 | 0 | Tr |
| Chocolate, regular | 1 Tbsp | 50 | 11 | 1 | 10 | 1 | Tr |
| Chocolate, light | 1 Tbsp | 25 | 7 | Tr | 7 | Tr | Tr |
| Cream, Whipped Topping | | | | | | | |
| Light cream | 1 cup | 700 | 7 | 0 | 7 | 5 | 75 |
| *Light cream* | *1 Tbsp* | *45* | *Tr* | *0* | *Tr* | *Tr* | *5* |
| Heavy cream | 1 cup | 820 | 7 | 0 | 7 | 5 | 88 |
| *Heavy cream* | *1 Tbsp* | *50* | *Tr* | *0* | *Tr* | *Tr* | *6* |
| *Pressurized in can* | *1 Tbsp* | *8* | *Tr* | *0* | *Tr* | *Tr* | *1* |
| Marshmallow Topping | 1 Tbsp | 50 | 12 | Tr | 12 | Tr | Tr |
| Strawberry Topping | 1 Tbsp | 50 | 11 | Tr | 11 | 1 | Tr |
| Tortellini | | | | | | | |
| Cheese filling | 1 cup | 270 | 40 | 2 | 38 | 12 | 7 |

| | Serving Size | Calories (g) | Total Carbs(g) | Fiber (g) | Net Carbs(g) | Protein (g) | Fat (g) |
|---|---|---|---|---|---|---|---|
| Meat filling | 1 cup | 340 | 55 | 1 | 54 | 21 | 9 |
| Spinach filling | 1 cup | 235 | 30 | 2 | 28 | 12 | 5 |
| **Tortellini Salad** w/dressing | ¾ cup | 350 | 24 | 5 | 19 | 11 | 24 |
| **Tortilla, 6" dia, ready to cook** | | | | | | | |
| Corn | 1 | 60 | 12 | 1 | 11 | 1 | 1 |
| Flour | 1 | 105 | 18 | 1 | 17 | 3 | 2 |
| **Tortilla Chips** | | | | | | | |
| Regular | 1 oz | 140 | 18 | 2 | 16 | 2 | 7 |
| Lowfat, baked | 1 oz | 115 | 22 | 2 | 20 | 4 | 1 |
| Nacho flavor, regular | 1 oz | 140 | 18 | 2 | 16 | 2 | 7 |
| Nacho flavor, reduced fat, baked | 1 oz | 125 | 20 | 1 | 19 | 2 | 4 |
| (also see Corn Chips) | | | | | | | |
| **Tostada** | | | | | | | |
| Beef, bean, & cheese | 1 | 330 | 30 | 2 | 28 | 16 | 17 |
| Chicken & cheese | 1 | 250 | 26 | 1 | 25 | 15 | 11 |
| Guacamole | 1 | 180 | 16 | 1 | 15 | 6 | 12 |
| **Trail Mix** | | | | | | | |
| Regular w/raisins, nuts, seeds, & chocolate chips | 1 cup | 705 | 66 | 9 | 57 | 21 | 47 |
| Tropical dried fruit mix | 1 cup | 570 | 92 | 11 | 81 | 9 | 24 |
| **Tuna** – see Fish | ... | ... | . | . | . | . | . |
| **Tuna Dishes** | | | | | | | |
| Tuna & broccoli w/creamy sauce | 1 cup | 300 | 31 | 1 | 30 | 14 | 12 |
| Tuna & noodle casserole | 1 cup | 320 | 37 | 2 | 35 | 20 | 10 |
| Tuna & pasta w/cheese sauce | 1 cup | 300 | 36 | 1 | 35 | 14 | 11 |
| Tuna & pasta w/creamy sauce | 1 cup | 300 | 36 | 1 | 35 | 14 | 12 |
| Tuna au gratin | 1 cup | 310 | 36 | 1 | 35 | 14 | 12 |
| Tuna fettuccine alfredo | 1 cup | 310 | 32 | 1 | 31 | 14 | 14 |
| Tuna romanoff | 1 cup | 280 | 38 | 1 | 37 | 15 | 8 |
| Tuna tetrazzini | 1 cup | 310 | 33 | 1 | 32 | 17 | 12 |
| **Tuna Salad** | | | | | | | |
| Prep w/tuna in oil, regular mayo dressing, pickle relish | ½ cup | 190 | 9 | 0 | 9 | 16 | 10 |

| | Serving Size | Calories (g) | Total Carbs(g) | Fiber (g) | Net Carbs(g) | Protein (g) | Fat (g) |
|---|---|---|---|---|---|---|---|
| Prep w/ tuna in water, light mayo dressing, pickle relish | ½ cup | 130 | 6 | 0 | 6 | 15 | 5 |
| **TURKEY** | | | | | | | |
| Fried Turkey patty, battered | 3 oz | 250 | 14 | Tr | 14 | 12 | 15 |
| Roast Turkey | | | | | | | |
| *light & dark meat* | *3 oz* | *145* | *3* | *0* | *3* | *22* | *5* |
| *light meat only* | *3 oz* | *135* | *0* | *0* | *0* | *25* | *4* |
| *dark meat only* | *3 oz* | *160* | *0* | *0* | *0* | *25* | *6* |
| *Giblets, simmered, chopped* | *1 cup* | *240* | *3* | *0* | *3* | *39* | *7* |
| *Ground Turkey* | *4 oz* | *195* | *0* | *0* | *0* | *22* | *11* |
| *Neck, simmered* | *2 slices* | *275* | *0* | *0* | *0* | *41* | *11* |
| (Other Turkey Products, see: Bologna, Hot Dog, Salami, Sausage & specific entrées) | | | | | | | |
| Turkey & Gravy | | | | | | | |
| *Banquet entrée* | 1 meal | 140 | 6 | Tr | 6 | 8 | 9 |
| Turkey Dijon | | | | | | | |
| *Lean Cuisine entrée* | 1 meal | 280 | 21 | 1 | 20 | 26 | 10 |
| Turkey Tetrazzini | | | | | | | |
| *Stouffers entrée* | 1 meal | 360 | 33 | 1 | 32 | 19 | 17 |
| **Turmeric, ground** | *½ tsp* | *4* | *1* | *Tr* | *Tr* | *Tr* | *Tr* |
| **Turnip, sliced, cooked** | *½ cup* | *20* | *4* | *Tr* | *4* | *1* | *Tr* |
| **Turnip Greens, cooked** | *½ cup* | *16* | *3* | *Tr* | *3* | *1* | *Tr* |
| Turnover | | | | | | | |
| Apple or Cherry, large | 1 | 410 | 63 | 4 | 59 | 4 | 16 |
| Apple, small | 1 | 170 | 21 | 2 | 19 | 2 | 8 |
| Blueberry, small | 1 | 165 | 23 | 2 | 21 | 2 | 8 |
| Cherry, small | 1 | 175 | 21 | 2 | 19 | 2 | 8 |
| **Vanilla Extract** | *1 tsp* | *12* | *1* | *0* | *1* | *Tr* | *Tr* |
| Veal | | | | | | | |
| *Chop, loin, braised* | *3.5 oz* | *285* | *0* | *0* | *0* | *30* | *17* |
| *Cutlet, braised, lean & fat* | *3 oz* | *180* | *0* | *0* | *0* | *31* | *5* |

| | Serving Size | Calories (g) | Total Carbs(g) | Fiber (g) | Net Carbs(g) | Protein (g) | Fat (g) |
|---|---|---|---|---|---|---|---|
| *Liver, braised* | *3.5 oz* | *165* | *0* | *0* | *0* | *22* | *7* |
| *Rib, roasted, lean & fat* | *3.5 oz* | *250* | *0* | *0* | *0* | *24* | *13* |
| Veal Marsala, *Le Menu entrée* | 1 meal | 250 | 25 | 1 | 24 | 25 | 5 |
| Veal Parmagiana | | | | | | | |
| *Le Menu entrée* | 1 meal | 175 | 9 | Tr | 9 | 22 | 6 |
| *Morton entrée* | 1 meal | 280 | 30 | 1 | 29 | 8 | 13 |
| Vegetable Burger, broiled | 1 patty | 100 | 9 | 4 | 5 | 15 | 1 |
| Vegetables, mixed *(See specific listings for individual vegetables)* | | | | | | | |
| *Mixed, canned, drained, heated* | 1 cup | 80 | 15 | 5 | 10 | 4 | Tr |
| *Mixed, frozen, w/o sauce, heated* | | | | | | | |
| Small vegetables- peas, carrots, beans, corn | 1 cup | 105 | 21 | 5 | 16 | 5 | Tr |
| *Large vegetable cuts, broccoli, cauliflower, whole mushroom* | *1 cup* | *27* | *4* | *3* | *1* | *3* | *0* |
| *Large vegetable cuts prep w/ butter sauce* | *1 cup* | *107* | *4* | *3* | *1* | *3* | *9* |
| Vegetables, mixed, *Birdseye* | | | | | | | |
| French style | ¾ cup | 110 | 10 | 3 | 7 | 6 | 2 |
| Italian style | ½ cup | 100 | 11 | 3 | 8 | 2 | 6 |
| Japanese style | ½ cup | 90 | 10 | 3 | 7 | 2 | 5 |
| Mexican style | ½ cup | 140 | 24 | 3 | 21 | 5 | 5 |
| *Oriental style* | *½ cup* | *60* | *4* | *2* | *2* | *2* | *4* |
| Vinegar | | | | | | | |
| *Regular* | *1 Tbsp* | *2* | *1* | *0* | *1* | *0* | *0* |
| *Cider vinegar* | *1 Tbsp* | *2* | *1* | *0* | *1* | *0* | *0* |
| Waffle | | | | | | | |
| Regular, prep from recipe, 7" dia | 1 piece | 215 | 25 | 1 | 24 | 6 | 11 |

| | Serving Size | Calories (g) | Total Carbs(g) | Fiber (g) | Net Carbs(g) | Protein (g) | Fat (g) |
|---|---|---|---|---|---|---|---|
| Frozen, toaster size, 4" dia | 1 piece | 90 | 13 | 1 | 12 | 2 | 3 |
| Lowfat, toaster size, 4" dia | 1 piece | 80 | 15 | Tr | 15 | 2 | 1 |
| **Walnut** – see Nuts | | | | | | | |
| **Water Chestnut,** canned, slices | 1 cup | 75 | 17 | 4 | 13 | 1 | Tr |
| ***Watercress, raw*** | *1/4 cup* | *2* | *Tr* | *Tr* | *Tr* | *Tr* | *0* |
| **Watermelon** | | | | | | | |
| Fresh, diced | 1 cup | 50 | 11 | 1 | 10 | 1 | 1 |
| Fresh, wedge, 1" thick, 1/16 of melon | | | | | | | |
| 15" long x 7 ½" dia | 1 wedge | 92 | 21 | 1 | 20 | 2 | 1 |
| ***Wheat Bran*** | *¼ cup* | *25* | *3* | *1* | *2* | *2* | *1* |
| ***Wheat Germ,*** *toasted, plain* | *1 Tbsp* | *27* | *3* | *1* | *2* | *2* | *1* |
| **Whipped Cream** – see Cream | ... | ... | . | . | . | . | . |
| **Wiener** – see Hot Dog | ... | ... | . | . | . | . | . |
| **Yam** – see Sweet Potato | ... | ... | . | . | . | . | . |
| ***Yeast*** | | | | | | | |
| ***Compressed*** | *1 cake* | *18* | *3* | *1* | *2* | *1* | *Tr* |
| ***Dry, active,*** *regular size pkg* | *1 pkg* | *21* | *3* | *2* | *1* | *3* | *Tr* |
| ***Dry, active*** | *1 tsp* | *12* | *2* | *1* | *1* | *2* | *Tr* |
| **Yogurt** | | | | | | | |
| Chocolate, regular | ½ cup | 120 | 18 | 2 | 16 | 3 | 4 |
| Chocolate, fat free | ½ cup | 90 | 17 | 1 | 16 | 5 | 0 |
| Strawberry, regular | ½ cup | 120 | 19 | Tr | 19 | 4 | 4 |
| Strawberry, fat free | ½ cup | 100 | 23 | 0 | 23 | 3 | 0 |
| Vanilla, regular | ½ cup | 120 | 18 | 0 | 18 | 3 | 4 |
| Vanilla, fat free | ½ cup | 110 | 23 | 0 | 23 | 4 | 0 |
| Yogurt, plain, made w/ whole milk | ½ cup | 140 | 11 | 0 | 11 | 8 | 7 |
| made w/ lowfat milk | ½ cup | 130 | 19 | 0 | 19 | 11 | 3 |
| made w/ skim milk | ½ cup | 120 | 15 | 0 | 15 | 13 | 0 |
| Yogurt w/fruit, regular varieties | ½ cup | 135 | 20 | 1 | 19 | 5 | 3 |

| | Serving Size | Calories (g) | Total Carbs(g) | Fiber (g) | Net Carbs(g) | Protein (g) | Fat (g) |
|---|---|---|---|---|---|---|---|
| Yogurt, w/fruit flavor, sugar-free | ½ cup | 95 | 16 | 0 | 16 | 9 | Tr |
| **Ziti w/ Meat Sauce** | | | | | | | |
| *Swanson entrée* | 1 meal | 560 | 58 | 1 | 57 | 28 | 23 |
| **Zucchini** | | | | | | | |
| ***Fresh, avg size*** | *1* | *5* | *1* | *Tr* | *Tr* | *Tr* | *0* |
| ***Sliced, cooked*** | *½ cup* | *15* | *4* | *1* | *3* | *Tr* | *0* |
| Breaded, fried | ½ cup | 165 | 16 | 2 | 14 | 4 | 9 |

## FAST FOOD RESTAURANTS

(See other Foods and Beverages listed separately)

| | Serving Size | Calories (g) | Total Carbs(g) | Fiber (g) | Net Carbs(g) | Protein (g) | Fat (g) |
|---|---|---|---|---|---|---|---|
| **Arby's** | | | | | | | |
| Apple turnover | 1 | 330 | 48 | 0 | 48 | 4 | 14 |
| Arby-Q | 1 | 430 | 48 | 3 | 45 | 22 | 18 |
| Arby's melt w/ cheddar | 1 | 370 | 36 | 2 | 34 | 18 | 18 |
| *Arby's sauce* | *1 svg* | *15* | *4* | *0* | *4* | *Tr* | *Tr* |
| Bacon cheddar deluxe | 1 | 540 | 38 | 3 | 35 | 22 | 34 |
| Baked potato, deluxe | 1 | 735 | 86 | 7 | 79 | 19 | 36 |
| Baked potato, plain | 1 | 355 | 82 | 7 | 75 | 7 | Tr |
| w/sour cream | 1 | 580 | 85 | 7 | 78 | 9 | 24 |
| Broccoli & cheddar | 1 | 580 | 89 | 9 | 80 | 14 | 20 |
| Barbecue sauce | 1 svg | 30 | 7 | 0 | 7 | 0 | 0 |
| Beef & cheddar sandwich | 1 | 490 | 40 | 2 | 38 | 25 | 28 |
| *Beefstock Au Jus* | *1* | *10* | *1* | *0* | *1* | *0* | *0* |
| Biscuit, plain | 1 | 280 | 34 | 1 | 33 | 6 | 15 |
| *Bleu cheese dressing* | *1 svg* | *290* | *2* | *0* | *2* | *2* | *31* |
| Blueberry muffin | 1 | 230 | 35 | 0 | 35 | 2 | 9 |
| Boston clam chowder | 1 svg | 190 | 18 | 1 | 17 | 9 | 9 |
| Breaded chicken fillet | 1 | 542 | 46 | 5 | 41 | 28 | 28 |
| Butterfinger polar swirl | 1 | 455 | 62 | 0 | 62 | 15 | 18 |
| *Cheddar cheese sauce* | *1 svg* | *35* | *1* | *0* | *1* | *1* | *3* |
| Cheddar curly fries | 1 svg | 335 | 40 | 3 | 37 | 3 | 18 |
| Cheesecake, plain | 1 | 320 | 23 | 1 | 22 | 5 | 23 |
| Cherry turnover | 1 | 320 | 46 | 1 | 45 | 4 | 13 |
| Chicken Cordon Bleu | 1 | 625 | 46 | 5 | 41 | 38 | 33 |
| Chicken fingers, 2 pieces/svg | 1 svg | 290 | 20 | 1 | 19 | 16 | 16 |
| Chocolate chip cookie | 1 | 125 | 16 | Tr | 16 | 2 | 6 |

| | Serving Size | Calories (g) | Total Carbs(g) | Fiber (g) | Net Carbs(g) | Protein (g) | Fat (g) |
|---|---|---|---|---|---|---|---|
| Chocolate shake | med | 450 | 76 | 0 | 76 | 15 | 12 |
| Cinnamon nut Danish | 1 | 360 | 60 | 1 | 59 | 6 | 11 |
| Cream of broccoli soup | 1 svg | 160 | 15 | 2 | 13 | 7 | 8 |
| Croissant, plain | 1 | 220 | 25 | 0 | 25 | 4 | 12 |
| Curly fries | 1 svg | 300 | 38 | 0 | 38 | 4 | 15 |
| Fish fillet | 1 | 530 | 50 | 2 | 48 | 23 | 27 |
| French dip | 1 svg | 475 | 40 | 3 | 37 | 30 | 22 |
| French fries | 1 | 240 | 30 | 3 | 27 | 2 | 13 |
| French toast stix, 6 pieces/svg | 1 svg | 430 | 52 | 3 | 49 | 10 | 21 |
| Garden salad w/o dressing | 1 | 60 | 12 | 5 | 7 | 3 | Tr |
| Giant roast beef | 1 | 555 | 43 | 5 | 38 | 35 | 28 |
| Grilled chicken deluxe | 1 | 430 | 41 | 3 | 38 | 23 | 20 |
| Grilled chicken barbecue | 1 | 390 | 47 | 2 | 45 | 23 | 13 |
| Ham & cheese | 1 | 355 | 24 | 2 | 22 | 24 | 14 |
| Ham & cheese melt | 1 | 335 | 34 | 2 | 32 | 20 | 13 |
| Heath polar swirl | 1 | 545 | 76 | 0 | 76 | 15 | 22 |
| Honey French dressing | 1 svg | 275 | 18 | 0 | 18 | 0 | 23 |
| *Horsey sauce* | *1 svg* | *55* | *2* | *0* | *2* | *0* | *5* |
| Hot ham & Swiss | 1 | 500 | 43 | 2 | 41 | 30 | 23 |
| Italian sub sandwich | 1 | 670 | 46 | 2 | 44 | 30 | 36 |
| *Italian sub sauce* | *1 svg* | *70* | *1* | *0* | *1* | *0* | *7* |
| Jamocha shake | small | 385 | 62 | 0 | 62 | 15 | 10 |
| Junior roast beef | 1 | 325 | 35 | 2 | 33 | 17 | 14 |
| *Light mayonnaise* | *1 svg* | *12* | *1* | *Tr* | *Tr* | *0* | *1* |
| Lumberjack mixed vegetables | 1 svg | 90 | 10 | 1 | 9 | 2 | 4 |
| Old fashion chicken noodle soup | 1 svg | 80 | 11 | 1 | 10 | 6 | 2 |
| Oreo polar swirl | 1 | 480 | 66 | 1 | 65 | 15 | 22 |

| | Serving Size | Calories (g) | Total Carbs(g) | Fiber (g) | Net Carbs(g) | Protein (g) | Fat (g) |
|---|---|---|---|---|---|---|---|
| *Parmesan cheese sauce* | *1 svg* | *70* | *1* | *0* | *1* | *0* | *7* |
| Peanut butter cup polar swirl | 1 | 515 | 61 | 1 | 60 | 20 | 24 |
| Philly beef & Swiss | 1 | 750 | 48 | 3 | 45 | 39 | 47 |
| Potato cakes | 1 svg | 200 | 20 | 2 | 18 | 2 | 12 |
| Potato with bacon soup | 1 svg | 170 | 23 | 2 | 21 | 6 | 7 |
| Red ranch dressing | 1 svg | 75 | 5 | 0 | 5 | 0 | 6 |
| *Reduced cal honey mayonnaise* | *1 svg* | *70* | *1* | *0* | *1* | *0* | *7* |
| *Reduced cal Italian dressing* | *1 svg* | *20* | *3* | *0* | *3* | *0* | *1* |
| Reduced cal buttermilk ranch | 1 svg | 50 | 12 | 0 | 12 | 0 | Tr |
| Roast beef sandwich, regular | 1 | 390 | 33 | 3 | 30 | 23 | 19 |
| Roast beef deluxe sandwich | 1 | 300 | 33 | 6 | 27 | 18 | 10 |
| Roast beef sub sandwich | 1 | 700 | 44 | 4 | 40 | 38 | 42 |
| Roast chicken club | 1 | 545 | 37 | 2 | 35 | 31 | 31 |
| Roast chicken Santa Fe | 1 | 435 | 35 | 1 | 34 | 29 | 22 |
| Roast chicken deluxe | 1 | 280 | 33 | 4 | 29 | 20 | 6 |
| Roast chicken salad | 1 | 150 | 12 | 5 | 7 | 20 | 2 |
| Roast turkey deluxe | 1 | 260 | 33 | 4 | 29 | 20 | 7 |
| *Side salad w/o dressing* | *1* | *25* | *4* | *2* | *2* | *1* | *Tr* |
| Snickers polar swirl | 1 | 510 | 73 | 1 | 72 | 15 | 19 |
| Super roast beef | 1 | 525 | 50 | 5 | 45 | 15 | 27 |
| *Tartar sauce* | *1 svg* | *140* | *0* | *0* | *0* | *0* | *15* |
| Thousand Island dressing | 1 svg | 260 | 7 | 0 | 7 | 0 | 26 |
| Timberline chili | 1 svg | 220 | 17 | 7 | 10 | 18 | 10 |
| Triple cheese melt | 1 | 720 | 46 | 2 | 44 | 37 | 45 |
| Turkey sub sandwich | 1 | 550 | 47 | 2 | 45 | 31 | 27 |
| Upper ten | 1 | 170 | 42 | 0 | 42 | 0 | 0 |

| | Serving Size | Calories (g) | Total Carbs (g) | Fiber (g) | Net Carbs (g) | Protein (g) | Fat (g) |
|---|---|---|---|---|---|---|---|
| Vanilla shake | small | 360 | 50 | 0 | 50 | 15 | 12 |
| Wisconsin cheese soup | 1 svg | 280 | 20 | 2 | 18 | 10 | 18 |
| **Baskin Robbins** | | | | | | | |
| *Ice Cream* | | | | | | | |
| Berries 'n Banana, no sugar added, lowfat | 4-oz scoop | 110 | 25 | 1 | 24 | 5 | 2 |
| Chocolate Chip | 4-oz scoop | 270 | 28 | 1 | 27 | 5 | 16 |
| Chocolate Chocolate Chip, sugarfree, lowfat | 4-oz scoop | 170 | 30 | 1 | 29 | 4 | 6 |
| Chocolate Chip Cookie Dough | 4-oz scoop | 290 | 36 | 1 | 35 | 5 | 15 |
| Chocolate | 4-oz scoop | 260 | 33 | 0 | 33 | 5 | 14 |
| Espresso & cream, lowfat | 4-oz scoop | 180 | 32 | 1 | 31 | 5 | 4 |
| Jamoca Almond Fudge | 4-oz scoop | 270 | 31 | 1 | 30 | 6 | 15 |
| Peanut Butter 'n Chocolate | 4-oz scoop | 320 | 31 | 1 | 30 | 7 | 20 |
| Rocky Road | 4-oz scoop | 290 | 36 | 1 | 35 | 5 | 15 |
| Vanilla | 4-oz scoop | 260 | 26 | 0 | 26 | 4 | 16 |
| Very Berry Strawberry | 4-oz scoop | 220 | 28 | 0 | 28 | 4 | 11 |
| *Yogurt* | | | | | | | |
| Butter Pecan, Truly Free | ½ cup | 90 | 17 | 1 | 16 | 4 | 0 |
| Café Mocha, Truly Free | ½ cup | 90 | 18 | 1 | 17 | 4 | 0 |
| Chocolate, nonfat, soft serve | ½ cup | 120 | 25 | 1 | 24 | 4 | 0 |
| Maui Brownie Madness, lowfat | 4-oz scoop | 210 | 39 | 1 | 38 | 6 | 4 |
| Peppermint, nonfat, soft serve | 4-oz scoop | 110 | 24 | 0 | 24 | 4 | 0 |
| Perils of Praline, lowfat | 4-oz scoop | 190 | 37 | 1 | 36 | 5 | 4 |
| Raspberry Cheese Louise, lowfat | 4-oz scoop | 190 | 37 | 1 | 36 | 5 | 4 |
| Vanilla, nonfat | 4-oz scoop | 150 | 32 | 0 | 32 | 6 | 0 |

| | Serving Size | Calories (g) | Total Carbs(g) | Fiber (g) | Net Carbs(g) | Protein (g) | Fat (g) |
|---|---|---|---|---|---|---|---|
| Vanilla, Truly Free | ½ cup | 90 | 17 | 1 | 16 | 4 | 0 |
| *Smoothies* | | | | | | | |
| Peach w/ yogurt | 16 oz | 360 | 83 | 3 | 80 | 8 | Tr |
| Strawberry Banana w/yogurt | 16 oz | 370 | 87 | 3 | 84 | 8 | 1 |
| Strawberry Banana w/yogurt | 16 oz | 380 | 93 | 3 | 90 | 5 | 1 |
| **Boston Market** | | | | | | | |
| Apples w/ cinnamon | 1 svg | 252 | 56 | 3 | 53 | Tr | 5 |
| Barbecue baked beans | 1 svg | 330 | 53 | 9 | 44 | 11 | 9 |
| Black beans with rice | 1 svg | 300 | 45 | 5 | 40 | 8 | 10 |
| Broccoli and rice casserole | 1svg | 240 | 26 | 3 | 23 | 5 | 12 |
| Brownie, chocolate | 1 | 310 | 51 | 3 | 48 | 3 | 10 |
| Cake, chocolate | 1 piece | 505 | 73 | 2 | 71 | 3 | 24 |
| Cake, hummingbird | 1 piece | 705 | 92 | 2 | 90 | 6 | 36 |
| Carrots, glazed | 1 svg | 280 | 35 | 2 | 33 | 1 | 15 |
| Cheesecake | 1 piece | 575 | 44 | 1 | 43 | 9 | 41 |
| *Chicken with skin, ½* | *1* | *625* | *2* | *0* | *2* | *70* | *37* |
| *Chicken w/o skin, ¼, dark meat* | *1* | *210* | *1* | *0* | *1* | *28* | *10* |
| *Chicken with skin, ¼, dark meat* | *1* | *325* | *2* | *0* | *2* | *30* | *22* |
| *Chicken w/o skin, ¼, white meat* | *1* | *165* | *1* | *0* | *1* | *31* | *4* |
| *Chicken w/ skin, ¼, white meat* | *1* | *310* | *2* | *0* | *2* | *43* | *17* |
| Chicken Caesar salad | 1 | 670 | 16 | 2 | 14 | 45 | 47 |
| Chicken pot pie | 1 | 745 | 57 | 3 | 54 | 26 | 46 |
| Chicken salad sandwich | 1 | 675 | 63 | 3 | 60 | 39 | 30 |
| Chicken sandwich | 1 | 390 | 60 | 2 | 58 | 31 | 5 |
| Chicken sandwich, barbecued | 1 | 540 | 84 | 2 | 82 | 30 | 9 |

| | Serving Size | Calories (g) | Total Carbs(g) | Fiber (g) | Net Carbs(g) | Protein (g) | Fat (g) |
|---|---|---|---|---|---|---|---|
| Chicken sandwich w/cheese | 1 | 630 | 61 | 2 | 59 | 37 | 28 |
| Cole slaw | 1 svg | 300 | 30 | 3 | 27 | 2 | 19 |
| Cookie, chocolate chip | 1 | 390 | 33 | 2 | 31 | 3 | 19 |
| Cookie, oatmeal | 1 | 390 | 47 | 2 | 45 | 5 | 20 |
| Cookie, peanut butter | 1 | 420 | 43 | 2 | 41 | 7 | 25 |
| Corn, buttered w/herbs | 1 svg | 180 | 30 | 2 | 28 | 5 | 4 |
| Corn, whole kernel | 1 svg | 180 | 30 | 2 | 28 | 5 | 4 |
| Cornbread | 1 svg | 200 | 33 | 2 | 31 | 3 | 6 |
| Cranberry relish | 1 svg | 330 | 70 | 2 | 68 | 1 | 5 |
| Cranberry walnut relish | 1 svg | 365 | 75 | 3 | 72 | 3 | 6 |
| *Green beans* | *1 svg* | *80* | *5* | *3* | *2* | *1* | *6* |
| Green bean casserole | 1 svg | 85 | 9 | 3 | 6 | 1 | 5 |
| Ham with honey glaze | 5 oz | 210 | 10 | 1 | 9 | 24 | 8 |
| Ham sandwich | 1 | 410 | 65 | 2 | 63 | 25 | 8 |
| Ham sandwich w/ cheese & sauce | 1 | 655 | 67 | 2 | 65 | 31 | 31 |
| Macaroni and cheese | 1 svg | 280 | 33 | 3 | 30 | 13 | 11 |
| Meatloaf | 5 oz | 290 | 15 | 1 | 14 | 20 | 17 |
| Meatloaf sandwich w/ cheese | 1 | 695 | 83 | 3 | 80 | 36 | 27 |
| Meatloaf sandwich, open faced | 1 | 730 | 74 | 2 | 72 | 29 | 36 |
| Pie, apple streusel | 1 piece | 480 | 63 | 2 | 61 | 4 | 18 |
| Pie, cherry streusel | 1 piece | 410 | 60 | 2 | 58 | 4 | 17 |
| Pie, pecan | 1 piece | 555 | 71 | 3 | 68 | 5 | 27 |
| Pie, pumpkin | 1 piece | 370 | 50 | 2 | 48 | 5 | 17 |
| Potatoes, dill & garlic | 1 svg | 130 | 25 | 2 | 23 | 3 | 3 |
| Potatoes, mashed | 1 svg | 185 | 25 | 2 | 23 | 3 | 8 |
| Potatoes, mashed w/gravy | 1 svg | 205 | 27 | 2 | 25 | 4 | 9 |
| Potatoes, new | 1 svg | 130 | 25 | 2 | 23 | 3 | 3 |
| Potato salad | 1 svg | 200 | 22 | 2 | 20 | 3 | 12 |

| | Serving Size | Calories (g) | Total Carbs(g) | Fiber (g) | Net Carbs(g) | Protein (g) | Fat (g) |
|---|---|---|---|---|---|---|---|
| Red beans and rice | 1 svg | 260 | 45 | 3 | 42 | 8 | 5 |
| Rice pilaf | 1 svg | 180 | 32 | 2 | 30 | 5 | 5 |
| Salad, Caesar | 1 svg | 200 | 7 | 2 | 5 | 7 | 17 |
| Salad, chunky chicken | 1 svg | 480 | 4 | 1 | 3 | 25 | 39 |
| Salad, cucumber | 1 svg | 120 | 9 | 3 | 6 | 2 | 10 |
| Salad, fruit | 1 svg | 70 | 15 | 3 | 12 | 1 | 1 |
| Salad, tortellini | 1 svg | 350 | 24 | 3 | 21 | 11 | 24 |
| Spinach, creamed | 1 svg | 260 | 11 | 3 | 8 | 9 | 20 |
| Squash, butternut | 1 svg | 160 | 25 | 3 | 22 | 2 | 6 |
| Squash casserole | 1 svg | 335 | 20 | 2 | 18 | 7 | 24 |
| Stuffing, savory | 1 svg | 310 | 44 | 2 | 42 | 6 | 12 |
| Sweet potato casserole | 1 svg | 280 | 39 | 3 | 36 | 3 | 18 |
| Turkey bacon club sandwich | 1 | 780 | 64 | 3 | 61 | 47 | 38 |
| *Turkey breast w/o skin* | *5 oz* | *170* | *1* | *0* | *1* | *36* | *1* |
| Turkey sandwich, regular | 1 | 390 | 61 | 2 | 59 | 33 | 4 |
| Turkey sandwich w/cheese | 1 | 615 | 64 | 2 | 62 | 39 | 25 |
| Turkey sandwich, open faced | 1 | 715 | 64 | 2 | 62 | 47 | 20 |
| *Vegetables, steamed, w/o sauce* | *1 svg* | *35* | *7* | *3* | *4* | *2* | *1* |
| Zucchini marinara | 1 svg | 80 | 10 | 2 | 8 | 2 | 4 |
| **Burger King** | | | | | | | |
| A.M. express dip | 1 svg | 85 | 21 | 2 | 19 | 2 | Tr |
| A.M. express grape jam | 1 svg | 30 | 7 | Tr | 7 | 0 | 0 |
| A.M. express strawberry jam | 1 svg | 30 | 8 | Tr | 8 | 0 | 0 |
| *Bacon bits* | *1 svg* | *15* | *0* | *0* | *0* | *1* | *1* |
| Barbecue sauce | 1 svg | 35 | 9 | 0 | 9 | 0 | Tr |
| Barbecue sauce, bull's eye | 1 svg | 20 | 5 | 0 | 5 | 0 | Tr |
| Biscuit with sausage | 1 | 585 | 41 | 1 | 40 | 16 | 40 |

| | Serving Size | Calories (g) | Total Carbs(g) | Fiber (g) | Net Carbs(g) | Protein (g) | Fat (g) |
|---|---|---|---|---|---|---|---|
| Biscuit w/ bacon, egg & cheese | 1 | 510 | 39 | 1 | 38 | 19 | 31 |
| BK big fish | 1 | 695 | 56 | 3 | 53 | 26 | 41 |
| BK broiler | 1 | 550 | 41 | 2 | 39 | 30 | 29 |
| *Bleu cheese dressing* | *1 svg* | *160* | *1* | *0* | *1* | *2* | *16* |
| *Broiled chicken salad* | *1* | *200* | *7* | *3* | *4* | *21* | *10* |
| Cheeseburger | 1 | 385 | 28 | 1 | 27 | 23 | 19 |
| Chicken sandwich | 1 | 705 | 54 | 2 | 52 | 26 | 43 |
| Chicken tenders, 8 pieces/svg | 1 svg | 310 | 19 | 3 | 16 | 3 | 17 |
| Chocolate shake | med | 445 | 84 | 2 | 82 | 2 | 7 |
| Croissanwich with sausage, egg & cheese | 1 | 600 | 25 | 1 | 24 | 1 | 46 |
| *Croutons* | *1 svg* | *30* | *4* | *0* | *4* | *Tr* | *1* |
| Double cheeseburger | 1 | 605 | 28 | 1 | 27 | 1 | 36 |
| Double cheeseburger w/ bacon | 1 | 640 | 28 | 1 | 27 | 1 | 39 |
| Double whopper | 1 | 875 | 45 | 3 | 42 | 3 | 56 |
| Double whopper w/ cheese | 1 | 965 | 46 | 3 | 43 | 3 | 63 |
| Dutch apple pie | 1 | 300 | 39 | 2 | 37 | 2 | 15 |
| French dressing | 1 svg | 145 | 11 | 0 | 11 | Tr | 10 |
| French fries | med | 375 | 43 | 3 | 40 | 3 | 20 |
| French fries, coated | med | 340 | 43 | 3 | 40 | 3 | 17 |
| French toast sticks | 1 svg | 505 | 60 | 1 | 59 | 1 | 27 |
| *Garden salad w/o dressing* | *1* | *100* | *7* | *3* | *4* | *3* | *5* |
| Hamburger | 1 | 335 | 28 | 1 | 27 | 1 | 15 |
| Hash browns | 1 | 220 | 25 | 2 | 23 | 2 | 12 |
| Honey dressing | 1 svg | 90 | 23 | Tr | 23 | Tr | Tr |
| *Land o'lakes classic whip blend* | *1 svg* | *65* | *0* | *0* | *0* | *0* | *7* |
| Onion rings | 1 svg | 315 | 41 | 6 | 35 | 6 | 14 |

| | Serving Size | Calories (g) | Total Carbs(g) | Fiber (g) | Net Carbs(g) | Protein (g) | Fat (g) |
|---|---|---|---|---|---|---|---|
| *Ranch dressing* | *1 svg* | *175* | *2* | *0* | *2* | *0* | *17* |
| *Reduced calorie Italian dressing* | *1 svg* | *15* | *3* | *0* | *3* | *0* | *1* |
| *Side salad w/o dressing* | *1* | *60* | *4* | *2* | *2* | *2* | *3* |
| Strawberry shake | med | 425 | 93 | 1 | 92 | 1 | 6 |
| Sweet & sour sauce | 1 svg | 45 | 11 | 0 | 11 | 0 | 0 |
| Tartar sauce | 1 svg | 145 | 7 | 0 | 7 | 0 | 12 |
| *Thousand Island dressing* | *1 svg* | *180* | *0* | *0* | *0* | *0* | *19* |
| Vanilla shake | med | 305 | 54 | 3 | 51 | 3 | 6 |
| Whopper junior | 1 | 425 | 29 | 2 | 27 | 2 | 24 |
| Whopper junior w/ cheese | 1 | 460 | 29 | 2 | 27 | 2 | 28 |
| Whopper | 1 | 645 | 45 | 3 | 42 | 3 | 38 |
| Whopper w/ cheese | 1 | 735 | 46 | 3 | 43 | 3 | 45 |
| Chinese Restaurant— see Panda Express Chinese Food | ... | ... | . | . | . | . | . |
| Dairy Queen | | | | | | | |
| *(all listings regular size, unless noted)* | | | | | | | |
| Banana split | 1 | 515 | 96 | 3 | 93 | 8 | 12 |
| Buster bar | 1 | 445 | 41 | 2 | 39 | 10 | 28 |
| Butterfinger blizzard | 1 | 750 | 115 | 1 | 114 | 16 | 26 |
| Caramel & nut bar | 1 | 260 | 32 | 1 | 31 | 5 | 13 |
| Chocolate cone | 1 | 360 | 56 | 1 | 55 | 9 | 11 |
| Chocolate soft serve | 1/2 cup | 150 | 22 | 1 | 21 | 4 | 5 |
| Chocolate dilly bar | 1 | 450 | 21 | 1 | 20 | 3 | 28 |
| Chocolate dilly bar, mint | 1 | 190 | 20 | 1 | 19 | 3 | 12 |
| Chocolate malt | 1 | 880 | 155 | 1 | 154 | 18 | 22 |
| Chocolate shake | 1 | 770 | 130 | 2 | 128 | 17 | 20 |
| Chocolate sundae | 1 | 410 | 73 | 1 | 72 | 8 | 10 |

| | Serving Size | Calories (g) | Total Carbs(g) | Fiber (g) | Net Carbs(g) | Protein (g) | Fat (g) |
|---|---|---|---|---|---|---|---|
| Cookie dough blizzard | 1 | 945 | 142 | 2 | 140 | 17 | 36 |
| Dipped cone | 1 | 515 | 63 | 1 | 62 | 9 | 25 |
| DQ frozen heart cake | 1 piece | 270 | 41 | 2 | 39 | 5 | 9 |
| DQ frozen log cake | 1 piece | 280 | 43 | 2 | 41 | 5 | 9 |
| DQ frozen round cake | 1 piece | 340 | 53 | 2 | 51 | 7 | 12 |
| DQ frozen sheet cake | 1 piece | 350 | 54 | 2 | 52 | 7 | 12 |
| DQ fudge bar | 1 | 60 | 13 | Tr | 13 | 3 | Tr |
| DQ lemon freez'r | 1 | 80 | 20 | Tr | 20 | 0 | 0 |
| DQ orange bar | 1 | 60 | 15 | Tr | 15 | Tr | 0 |
| DQ sandwich | 1 | 150 | 24 | 1 | 23 | 3 | 5 |
| DQ vanilla orange bar | 1 | 60 | 17 | Tr | 17 | 2 | 0 |
| DQ vanilla soft serve | ½ cup | 140 | 22 | Tr | 22 | 3 | 5 |
| DQ yogurt, nonfat frozen | ½ cup | 100 | 21 | Tr | 21 | 3 | 0 |
| Fudge nut bar | 1 | 410 | 40 | 2 | 38 | 8 | 25 |
| Heath blizzard | 1 | 818 | 119 | 2 | 117 | 14 | 33 |
| Heath breeze | 1 | 710 | 123 | 2 | 121 | 15 | 18 |
| Heath treatzza pizza | 1 slice | 180 | 28 | 2 | 26 | 3 | 7 |
| M&M treatzza pizza | 1 slice | 190 | 29 | 2 | 27 | 3 | 7 |
| Misty slush | 1 | 290 | 74 | Tr | 74 | 0 | 0 |
| Oreo blizzard | 1 | 640 | 79 | 2 | 77 | 10 | 23 |
| Peanut buster parfait | 1 | 730 | 99 | 2 | 97 | 16 | 31 |
| Peanut butter fudge treatzza pizza | 1 slice | 220 | 28 | 2 | 26 | 4 | 10 |
| Queen's choice choc. big scoop | 1 | 250 | 28 | 2 | 26 | 4 | 14 |
| Queen's choice vanilla big scoop | 1 | 250 | 27 | Tr | 27 | 4 | 14 |
| Reeses peanut butter cup blizzard | 1 | 785 | 105 | 2 | 103 | 19 | 33 |
| Starkiss | 1 | 80 | 21 | Tr | 21 | 0 | 0 |
| Strawberry banana treatzza pizza | 1 slice | 180 | 29 | 2 | 27 | 3 | 6 |

| | Serving Size | Calories (g) | Total Carbs (g) | Fiber (g) | Net Carbs (g) | Protein (g) | Fat (g) |
|---|---|---|---|---|---|---|---|
| Strawberry blizzard | 1 | 570 | 95 | 1 | 94 | 12 | 16 |
| Strawberry breeze | 1 | 460 | 99 | 1 | 98 | 13 | 1 |
| Strawberry misty cooler | 1 | 190 | 49 | Tr | 49 | 0 | 0 |
| Strawberry shortcake | 1 piece | 430 | 24 | 2 | 22 | 7 | 14 |
| Toffee dilly bar | 1 | 210 | 24 | 1 | 23 | 3 | 12 |
| Vanilla cone | 1 | 355 | 57 | 0 | 57 | 8 | 10 |
| Vanilla cone, small | 1 | 230 | 38 | 0 | 38 | 6 | 7 |
| Yogurt cone | 1 | 280 | 59 | 1 | 58 | 9 | 1 |
| Yogurt cup | 1 | 230 | 49 | 1 | 48 | 8 | 1 |
| Yogurt strawberry sundae | 1 | 305 | 66 | 1 | 65 | 10 | 1 |
| **Denny's** | | | | | | | |
| Banana split | 1 | 885 | 121 | 3 | 118 | 15 | 43 |
| Biscuit with sausage gravy | 7 oz | 395 | 45 | 2 | 43 | 8 | 21 |
| ***Buffalo wings, 12 per svg*** | *1 svg* | *855* | *1* | *Tr* | *Tr* | *92* | *54* |
| Carrots with honey glaze | 1 svg | 80 | 12 | 2 | 10 | 1 | 3 |
| Charleston chicken dinner | 1 | 325 | 16 | 1 | 15 | 25 | 18 |
| Cheesecake | 1 slice | 470 | 48 | Tr | 48 | 6 | 27 |
| Cheese fries with chili | 1 svg | 815 | 77 | 3 | 74 | 29 | 44 |
| Cheese fries, smothered | 1 svg | 765 | 69 | 3 | 66 | 27 | 48 |
| Chicken burger sandwich | 1 | 630 | 53 | 2 | 51 | 35 | 32 |
| Chicken burger buffalo sandwich | 1 | 800 | 67 | 2 | 65 | 37 | 45 |
| Chicken fried steak | 4 oz | 265 | 14 | 1 | 13 | 15 | 17 |
| Chicken strips, 5 per svg | 1 svg | 720 | 56 | 2 | 54 | 47 | 33 |
| Chicken strips buffalo, 5 per svg | 1 svg | 735 | 43 | 1 | 42 | 48 | 42 |
| Chili with cheese topping | 1 svg | 400 | 21 | 1 | 20 | 26 | 19 |
| Chocolate layer cake | 1 slice | 275 | 42 | 2 | 40 | 4 | 12 |
| Club sandwich | 1 | 720 | 62 | 2 | 60 | 32 | 38 |
| Corn with butter sauce | 1 svg | 120 | 19 | 2 | 17 | 3 | 4 |

| | Serving Size | Calories (g) | Total Carbs(g) | Fiber (g) | Net Carbs(g) | Protein (g) | Fat (g) |
|---|---|---|---|---|---|---|---|
| Country fried potatoes | 1 svg | 515 | 23 | 3 | 20 | 3 | 35 |
| Double scoop sundae | 1 | 375 | 29 | 1 | 28 | 6 | 27 |
| French fries | 1 svg | 260 | 35 | 3 | 32 | 5 | 12 |
| w/ seasoning | 1 svg | 320 | 44 | 4 | 40 | 5 | 14 |
| Fried shrimp dinner | 8 oz | 220 | 18 | 1 | 17 | 17 | 10 |
| Garden salad deluxe w/ chicken | 1 | 265 | 10 | 5 | 5 | 32 | 11 |
| Grasshopper blender blaster | 15 oz | 735 | 92 | 1 | 91 | 13 | 37 |
| Grasshopper sundae | 14 oz | 735 | 97 | 1 | 96 | 13 | 34 |
| ***Green beans w/ bacon*** | ***1 svg*** | ***60*** | ***6*** | ***2*** | ***4*** | ***1*** | ***4*** |
| Green peas w/ butter sauce | 1 svg | 100 | 14 | 3 | 11 | 5 | 2 |
| ***Grilled chicken dinner*** | ***1*** | ***130*** | ***0*** | ***0*** | ***0*** | ***24*** | ***4*** |
| Grilled chicken sandwich | 1 | 435 | 56 | 2 | 54 | 35 | 9 |
| Grilled chicken stir fried | 1 | 865 | 149 | 3 | 146 | 43 | 10 |
| ***Grilled salmon dinner*** | ***6 oz*** | ***210*** | ***1*** | ***0*** | ***1*** | ***43*** | ***4*** |
| Ham & Swiss sandwich | 1 | 535 | 40 | 2 | 38 | 23 | 31 |
| Hamburger, | | | | | | | |
| Bacon & cheddar | 1 | 875 | 58 | 2 | 56 | 53 | 52 |
| Big Texas BBQ | 1 | 930 | 53 | 2 | 51 | 53 | 58 |
| Boca | 1 | 615 | 66 | 2 | 64 | 29 | 28 |
| Classic | 1 | 675 | 42 | 2 | 40 | 37 | 40 |
| Classic doubledecker | 1 | 1375 | 81 | 3 | 78 | 62 | 92 |
| Classic w/cheese | 1 | 836 | 43 | 2 | 41 | 47 | 53 |
| Mushroom & Swiss | 1 | 872 | 58 | 2 | 56 | 48 | 51 |
| Hot fudge cake sundae | 1 svg | 620 | 73 | 2 | 71 | 7 | 35 |
| Malted milk shake, chocolate | 12 oz | 585 | 82 | 1 | 81 | 12 | 26 |
| Malted milk shake, vanilla | 12 oz | 585 | 82 | Tr | 82 | 12 | 26 |
| Mashed potatoes | 1 svg | 105 | 21 | 2 | 19 | 3 | 1 |
| Mashed potatoes w/ cheddar | 1 svg | 117 | 22 | 2 | 20 | 3 | 2 |
| Mozzarella sticks, 8 per svg | 1 svg | 710 | 49 | 1 | 48 | 36 | 41 |

| | Serving Size | Calories (g) | Total Carbs(g) | Fiber (g) | Net Carbs(g) | Protein (g) | Fat (g) |
|---|---|---|---|---|---|---|---|
| Onion rings | 1 svg | 380 | 38 | 2 | 36 | 5 | 23 |
| Peaches and cream sundae | 1 | 570 | 91 | 1 | 90 | 5 | 22 |
| Pie, | | | | | | | |
| Apple | 1 slice | 475 | 64 | 2 | 62 | 3 | 24 |
| Cherry | 1 slice | 630 | 101 | 3 | 98 | 3 | 25 |
| Chocolate peanut butter | 1 slice | 655 | 64 | 3 | 61 | 15 | 39 |
| Hershey's chocolate chip | 1 slice | 600 | 58 | 2 | 56 | 6 | 36 |
| Pie, Oreo cookies & cream | 1 slice | 650 | 67 | 2 | 65 | 6 | 40 |
| Pot roast dinner | 1 | 295 | 5 | Tr | 5 | 42 | 11 |
| Roast turkey dinner | 1 | 388 | 38 | 1 | 37 | 46 | 3 |
| Rueben sandwich | 1 | 580 | 37 | 2 | 35 | 27 | 35 |
| Shake, | | | | | | | |
| Chocolate | 12 oz | 560 | 76 | 1 | 75 | 11 | 26 |
| Vanilla | 12 oz | 560 | 76 | Tr | 76 | 11 | 26 |
| *Shrimp scampi skillet dinner* | *1 svg* | *290* | *3* | *Tr* | *3* | *25* | *19* |
| *Sirloin steak dinner* | *8 oz* | *340* | *1* | *0* | *1* | *18* | *28* |
| Slim slam | 12 oz | 495 | 98 | 1 | 97 | 34 | 12 |
| Steak and shrimp dinner | 9 oz | 640 | 31 | 1 | 30 | 36 | 42 |
| Super bird sandwich | 1 | 620 | 48 | 2 | 46 | 35 | 32 |
| *T-bone steak dinner* | *14 oz* | *860* | *0* | *0* | *0* | *65* | *65* |
| *Two egg breakfast* | *1* | *825* | *1* | *0* | *1* | *6* | *67* |
| Turkey breast sandwich | 1 | 475 | 39 | 2 | 37 | 23 | 26 |
| Vegetable rice pilaf | 1 svg | 85 | 16 | 2 | 14 | 2 | 1 |
| Western wings roundup | 20 oz | 1515 | 89 | 3 | 86 | 89 | 88 |

| | Serving Size | Calories (g) | Total Carbs(g) | Fiber (g) | Net Carbs(g) | Protein (g) | Fat (g) |
|---|---|---|---|---|---|---|---|
| **Domino's Pizza** | | | | | | | |
| *(1 slice = ⅛ Pizza)* | | | | | | | |
| Feast Pizzas, Med | 12-inch | | | | | | |
| *America's favorite* | | | | | | | |
|   Classic hand-tossed | 1 slice | 255 | 29 | 2 | 27 | 10 | 12 |
|   Crunchy thin crust | 1 slice | 210 | 15 | 1 | 14 | 8 | 14 |
|   Ultimate deep dish | 1 slice | 310 | 29 | 2 | 27 | 12 | 17 |
| *Bacon cheeseburger* | | | | | | | |
|   Classic hand-tossed | 1 slice | 275 | 28 | 2 | 26 | 12 | 13 |
|   Crunchy thin crust | 1 slice | 225 | 14 | 1 | 13 | 10 | 15 |
|   Ultimate deep dish | 1 slice | 325 | 28 | 2 | 26 | 14 | 19 |
| *Barbecue* | | | | | | | |
|   Classic hand-tossed | 1 slice | 250 | 31 | 1 | 30 | 11 | 10 |
|   Crunchy thin crust | 1 slice | 205 | 17 | 1 | 16 | 8 | 12 |
|   Ultimate deep dish | 1 slice | 304 | 32 | 2 | 30 | 12 | 15 |
| *Deluxe* | | | | | | | |
|   Classic hand-tossed | 1 slice | 235 | 29 | 2 | 27 | 9 | 10 |
|   Crunchy thin crust | 1 slice | 185 | 15 | 1 | 14 | 7 | 12 |
|   Ultimate deep dish | 1 slice | 285 | 29 | 2 | 27 | 11 | 15 |
| *Extravaganzza* | | | | | | | |
|   Classic hand-tossed | 1 slice | 290 | 30 | 2 | 28 | 13 | 14 |
|   Crunchy thin crust | 1 slice | 240 | 16 | 1 | 15 | 11 | 16 |
|   Ultimate deep dish | 1 slice | 340 | 30 | 2 | 28 | 14 | 20 |
| *Hawaiian* | | | | | | | |
|   Classic hand-tossed | 1 slice | 225 | 30 | 2 | 28 | 10 | 8 |
|   Crunchy thin crust | 1 slice | 175 | 16 | 1 | 15 | 8 | 10 |
|   Ultimate deep dish | 1 slice | 275 | 30 | 2 | 28 | 12 | 13 |
| *Meatzza* | | | | | | | |
|   Classic hand-tossed | 1 slice | 281 | 29 | 2 | 27 | 13 | 14 |
|   Crunchy thin crust | 1 slice | 232 | 15 | 1 | 14 | 11 | 15 |
|   Ultimate deep dish | 1 slice | 335 | 29 | 2 | 27 | 14 | 19 |
| *Pepperoni* | | | | | | | |
|   Classic hand-tossed | 1 slice | 265 | 28 | 2 | 26 | 11 | 13 |
|   Crunchy thin crust | 1 slice | 215 | 14 | 1 | 13 | 9 | 14 |
|   Ultimate deep dish | 1 slice | 320 | 29 | 2 | 27 | 13 | 18 |
| *Veggie* | | | | | | | |
|   Classic hand-tossed | 1 slice | 220 | 29 | 2 | 27 | 9 | 8 |
|   Crunchy thin crust | 1 slice | 170 | 15 | 1 | 14 | 7 | 10 |

| | Serving Size | Calories (g) | Total Carbs(g) | Fiber (g) | Net Carbs(g) | Protein (g) | Fat (g) |
|---|---|---|---|---|---|---|---|
| Ultimate deep dish | 1 slice | 270 | 30 | 2 | 28 | 11 | 14 |
| **Feast Pizzas, Lg** | 14-inch | | | | | | |
| *America's favorite* | | | | | | | |
| Classic hand-tossed | 1 slice | 355 | 39 | 2 | 37 | 14 | 16 |
| Crunchy thin crust | 1 slice | 285 | 20 | 2 | 18 | 11 | 19 |
| Ultimate deep dish | 1 slice | 435 | 42 | 3 | 39 | 17 | 24 |
| *Bacon cheeseburger* | | | | | | | |
| Classic hand-tossed | 1 slice | 380 | 38 | 2 | 36 | 17 | 18 |
| Crunchy thin crust | 1 slice | 310 | 19 | 1 | 18 | 14 | 21 |
| Ultimate deep dish | 1 slice | 460 | 41 | 2 | 39 | 20 | 26 |
| *Barbecue* | | | | | | | |
| Classic hand-tossed | 1 slice | 345 | 43 | 2 | 41 | 14 | 14 |
| Crunchy thin crust | 1 slice | 275 | 24 | 1 | 23 | 11 | 16 |
| Ultimate deep dish | 1 slice | 425 | 46 | 2 | 44 | 17 | 21 |
| *Deluxe* | | | | | | | |
| Classic hand-tossed | 1 slice | 315 | 39 | 2 | 37 | 13 | 13 |
| Crunchy thin crust | 1 slice | 245 | 20 | 2 | 18 | 10 | 15 |
| Ultimate deep dish | 1 slice | 395 | 42 | 3 | 39 | 15 | 20 |
| *Extravaganza* | | | | | | | |
| Classic hand-tossed | 1 slice | 388 | 40 | 3 | 37 | 17 | 19 |
| Crunchy thin crust | 1 slice | 320 | 21 | 2 | 19 | 14 | 26 |
| Ultimate deep dish | 1 slice | 470 | 43 | 3 | 40 | 20 | 19 |
| *Hawaiian* | | | | | | | |
| Classic hand-tossed | 1 slice | 310 | 41 | 2 | 39 | 14 | 11 |
| Crunchy thin crust | 1 slice | 240 | 43 | 2 | 41 | 11 | 13 |
| Ultimate deep dish | 1 slice | 390 | 21 | 3 | 18 | 17 | 18 |
| *Meatzza* | | | | | | | |
| Classic hand-tossed | 1 slice | 380 | 39 | 2 | 37 | 17 | 18 |
| Crunchy thin crust | 1 slice | 310 | 20 | 2 | 18 | 14 | 20 |
| Ultimate deep dish | 1 slice | 458 | 42 | 3 | 39 | 19 | 25 |
| *Pepperoni* | | | | | | | |
| Classic hand-tossed | 1 slice | 360 | 39 | 2 | 37 | 16 | 17 |
| Crunchy thin crust | 1 slice | 295 | 20 | 1 | 19 | 13 | 19 |
| Ultimate deep dish | 1 slice | 440 | 42 | 3 | 39 | 18 | 24 |
| *Veggie* | | | | | | | |
| Classic hand-tossed | 1 slice | 300 | 40 | 3 | 37 | 13 | 11 |
| Crunchy thin crust | 1 slice | 230 | 43 | 2 | 41 | 10 | 14 |
| Ultimate deep dish | 1 slice | 380 | 21 | 3 | 18 | 15 | 18 |

| | Serving Size | Calories (g) | Total Carbs(g) | Fiber (g) | Net Carbs(g) | Protein (g) | Fat (g) |
|---|---|---|---|---|---|---|---|
| Med 12-inch Pizzas (reg, not Feast pizza) | | | | | | | |
| *Cheese* | | | | | | | |
| Classic hand-tossed | 1 slice | 185 | 28 | 1 | 27 | 7 | 6 |
| Crunchy thin crust | 1 slice | 135 | 14 | 1 | 13 | 5 | 7 |
| Ultimate deep dish | 1 slice | 240 | 28 | 2 | 26 | 9 | 11 |
| *Beef* | | | | | | | |
| Classic hand-tossed | 1 slice | 225 | 28 | 2 | 26 | 9 | 9 |
| Crunchy thin crust | 1 slice | 175 | 14 | 1 | 13 | 7 | 11 |
| Ultimate deep dish | 1 slice | 277 | 28 | 2 | 26 | 11 | 15 |
| *Green pepper, mushroom, onion* | | | | | | | |
| Classic hand-tossed | 1 slice | 190 | 29 | 2 | 27 | 8 | 6 |
| Crunchy thin crust | 1 slice | 142 | 15 | 1 | 14 | 6 | 8 |
| Ultimate deep dish | 1 slice | 244 | 30 | 2 | 28 | 9 | 11 |
| *Ham* | | | | | | | |
| Classic hand-tossed | 1 slice | 195 | 28 | 1 | 27 | 9 | 6 |
| Crunchy thin crust | 1 slice | 150 | 14 | 1 | 13 | 7 | 8 |
| Ultimate deep dish | 1 slice | 250 | 28 | 2 | 26 | 11 | 12 |
| *Ham & pineapple* | | | | | | | |
| Classic hand-tossed | 1 slice | 200 | 29 | 2 | 27 | 9 | 6 |
| Crunchy thin crust | 1 slice | 150 | 15 | 1 | 14 | 7 | 8 |
| Ultimate deep dish | 1 slice | 250 | 30 | 2 | 28 | 10 | 12 |
| *Pepperoni* | | | | | | | |
| Classic hand-tossed | 1 slice | 223 | 28 | 2 | 26 | 9 | 9 |
| Crunchy thin crust | 1 slice | 175 | 14 | 1 | 13 | 7 | 11 |
| Ultimate deep dish | 1 slice | 275 | 28 | 2 | 26 | 11 | 14 |
| *Pepperoni & sausage* | | | | | | | |
| Classic hand-tossed | 1 slice | 255 | 28 | 2 | 26 | 10 | 12 |
| Crunchy thin crust | 1 slice | 206 | 14 | 1 | 13 | 8 | 14 |
| Ultimate deep dish | 1 slice | 307 | 29 | 2 | 27 | 12 | 17 |
| *Sausage* | | | | | | | |
| Classic hand-tossed | 1 slice | 230 | 28 | 2 | 26 | 9 | 10 |
| Crunchy thin crust | 1 slice | 181 | 14 | 1 | 13 | 7 | 11 |
| Ultimate deep dish | 1 slice | 283 | 29 | 2 | 27 | 11 | 15 |

| | Serving Size | Calories (g) | Total Carbs(g) | Fiber (g) | Net Carbs(g) | Protein (g) | Fat (g) |
|---|---|---|---|---|---|---|---|
| **Lg 14-inch Pizzas (regular, not Feast pizza)** | | | | | | | |
| *Cheese* | | | | | | | |
| Classic hand-tossed | 1 slice | 256 | 38 | 2 | 36 | 10 | 8 |
| Crunchy thin crust | 1 slice | 190 | 19 | 1 | 18 | 7 | 10 |
| Ultimate deep dish | 1 slice | 336 | 41 | 2 | 39 | 13 | 15 |
| *Beef* | | | | | | | |
| Classic hand-tossed | 1 slice | 310 | 38 | 2 | 36 | 13 | 13 |
| Crunchy thin crust | 1 slice | 243 | 19 | 1 | 18 | 10 | 15 |
| Ultimate deep dish | 1 slice | 390 | 41 | 2 | 39 | 15 | 20 |
| *Green pepper, mushroom, onion* | | | | | | | |
| Classic hand-tossed | 1 slice | 263 | 39 | 2 | 37 | 11 | 8 |
| Crunchy thin crust | 1 slice | 200 | 21 | 2 | 19 | 8 | 10 |
| Ultimate deep dish | 1 slice | 343 | 42 | 3 | 39 | 13 | 15 |
| *Ham* | | | | | | | |
| Classic hand-tossed | 1 slice | 270 | 38 | 2 | 36 | 12 | 9 |
| Crunchy thin crust | 1 slice | 204 | 19 | 1 | 18 | 9 | 11 |
| Ultimate deep dish | 1 slice | 350 | 41 | 2 | 39 | 15 | 16 |
| *Ham & pineapple* | | | | | | | |
| Classic hand-tossed | 1 slice | 275 | 40 | 2 | 38 | 12 | 9 |
| Crunchy thin crust | 1 slice | 207 | 21 | 1 | 20 | 9 | 11 |
| Ultimate deep dish | 1 slice | 355 | 42 | 2 | 40 | 14 | 16 |
| *Pepperoni* | | | | | | | |
| Classic hand-tossed | 1 slice | 305 | 38 | 2 | 36 | 12 | 12 |
| Crunchy thin crust | 1 slice | 237 | 19 | 1 | 18 | 10 | 15 |
| Ultimate deep dish | 1 slice | 385 | 41 | 2 | 39 | 15 | 20 |
| *Pepperoni & sausage* | | | | | | | |
| Classic hand-tossed | 1 slice | 350 | 39 | 2 | 37 | 14 | 16 |
| Crunchy thin crust | 1 slice | 282 | 19 | 2 | 17 | 11 | 19 |
| Ultimate deep dish | 1 slice | 430 | 41 | 3 | 38 | 17 | 23 |
| *Sausage* | | | | | | | |
| Classic hand-tossed | 1 slice | 320 | 39 | 2 | 37 | 13 | 14 |
| Crunchy thin crust | 1 slice | 250 | 20 | 2 | 18 | 10 | 16 |
| Ultimate deep dish | 1 slice | 400 | 42 | 3 | 39 | 15 | 21 |
| **Side Orders & Condiments** | | | | | | | |
| ***Barbecue buffalo wings*** | **1 piece** | **50** | **2** | **0** | **2** | **6** | **3** |

| | Serving Size | Calories (g) | Total Carbs(g) | Fiber (g) | Net Carbs(g) | Protein (g) | Fat (g) |
|---|---|---|---|---|---|---|---|
| *Blue cheese dipping sauce* | *1 svg* | *225* | *2* | *0* | *2* | *1* | *24* |
| Bread sticks | 1 piece | 115 | 12 | 0 | 12 | 2 | 6 |
| *Buffalo chicken kickers* | *1 piece* | *47* | *3* | *0* | *3* | *4* | *2* |
| Cheesy bread | 1 piece | 125 | 13 | 0 | 13 | 4 | 7 |
| Cinnamon stix | 1 piece | 125 | 15 | 1 | 14 | 2 | 6 |
| *Garlic sauce* | *1 svg* | *440* | *0* | *0* | *0* | *0* | *49* |
| *Hot buffalo wings* | *1 piece* | *45* | *1* | *0* | *1* | *5* | *3* |
| *Hot dipping sauce* | *1 svg* | *15* | *4* | *0* | *4* | *0* | *0* |
| Marinara dipping sauce | 1 svg | 25 | 5 | 0 | 5 | 1 | Tr |
| *Ranch dipping sauce* | *1 svg* | *195* | *2* | *0* | *2* | *1* | *21* |
| Sweet icing | 1 svg | 250 | 57 | 0 | 57 | 0 | 3 |
| **Dunkin' Donuts** | | | | | | | |
| Bagels | | | | | | | |
| Berry berry | 1 | 345 | 69 | 4 | 65 | 11 | 3 |
| Blueberry | 1 | 350 | 69 | 4 | 65 | 11 | 3 |
| Cinnamon raisin | 1 | 335 | 65 | 3 | 62 | 10 | 3 |
| Everything | 1 | 430 | 75 | 3 | 72 | 17 | 7 |
| Garlic | 1 | 410 | 79 | 3 | 76 | 16 | 4 |
| Onion | 1 | 375 | 71 | 4 | 67 | 14 | 4 |
| Plain | 1 | 360 | 69 | 2 | 67 | 14 | 3 |
| Poppyseed | 1 | 440 | 72 | 3 | 69 | 17 | 10 |
| Salt | 1 | 360 | 69 | 2 | 67 | 14 | 3 |
| Sesame | 1 | 455 | 71 | 3 | 68 | 18 | 11 |
| Sourdough | 1 | 340 | 65 | 2 | 63 | 15 | 3 |
| Wheat | 1 | 350 | 66 | 4 | 62 | 13 | 5 |
| Cream cheese | | | | | | | |
| *Chive* | *2 oz* | *170* | *4* | *2* | *2* | *4* | *17* |
| *Garden vegetable* | *2 oz* | *170* | *4* | *0* | *4* | *2* | *15* |
| Light | 2 oz | 110 | 6 | 0 | 6 | 4 | 9 |
| *Plain* | *2 oz* | *190* | *4* | *0* | *4* | *4* | *17* |
| *Salmon* | *2 oz* | *170* | *2* | *0* | *2* | *4* | *17* |
| *Shedd's buttermatch blend* | *1 Tbsp* | *80* | *0* | *0* | *0* | *0* | *9* |
| Strawberry | 2 oz | 195 | 9 | 0 | 9 | 4 | 17 |

| | Serving Size | Calories (g) | Total Carbs(g) | Fiber (g) | Net Carbs(g) | Protein (g) | Fat (g) |
|---|---|---|---|---|---|---|---|
| **Cookies** | | | | | | | |
| Chocolate chunk | 1 | 220 | 28 | 1 | 27 | 3 | 11 |
| Chocolate chunk w/ walnuts | 1 | 230 | 27 | 1 | 26 | 3 | 12 |
| Oatmeal raisin pecan | 1 | 220 | 29 | 1 | 28 | 3 | 10 |
| White chocolate chunk | 1 | 235 | 28 | 1 | 27 | 3 | 12 |
| **Danish** | | | | | | | |
| Apple | 1 | 250 | 36 | 0 | 36 | 4 | 10 |
| Cheese | 1 | 275 | 32 | 0 | 32 | 4 | 14 |
| Strawberry cheese | 1 | 250 | 33 | 0 | 33 | 4 | 12 |
| **Donuts** | | | | | | | |
| Apple crumb | 1 | 235 | 34 | 1 | 33 | 3 | 10 |
| Apple & spice | 1 | 200 | 29 | 1 | 28 | 3 | 8 |
| Bavarian kreme | 1 | 210 | 30 | 1 | 29 | 3 | 9 |
| Black raspberry | 1 | 210 | 32 | 1 | 31 | 3 | 8 |
| Blueberry cake | 1 | 290 | 35 | 1 | 34 | 3 | 16 |
| Blueberry crumb | 1 | 240 | 36 | 1 | 35 | 3 | 10 |
| Boston kreme | 1 | 240 | 36 | 1 | 35 | 3 | 9 |
| Chocolate coconut cake | 1 | 300 | 31 | 1 | 30 | 4 | 19 |
| Chocolate-frosted cake | 1 | 360 | 40 | 1 | 39 | 4 | 20 |
| Chocolate-frosted | 1 | 200 | 29 | 1 | 28 | 3 | 9 |
| Chocolate-glazed cake | 1 | 295 | 33 | 1 | 32 | 3 | 16 |
| Chocolate kreme-filled | 1 | 270 | 35 | 1 | 34 | 3 | 13 |
| Cinnamon cake | 1 | 330 | 34 | 1 | 33 | 4 | 20 |
| Double chocolate cake | 1 | 310 | 39 | 2 | 37 | 3 | 17 |
| French cruller | 1 | 150 | 17 | 1 | 16 | 2 | 8 |
| Glazed cake | 1 | 350 | 41 | 1 | 40 | 4 | 19 |
| Glazed | 1 | 180 | 25 | 1 | 24 | 3 | 8 |
| Jelly-filled | 1 | 210 | 32 | 1 | 31 | 3 | 8 |
| Maple-frosted | 1 | 210 | 30 | 1 | 29 | 3 | 9 |
| Marble-frosted | 1 | 200 | 29 | 1 | 28 | 3 | 9 |
| Old fashioned cake | 1 | 300 | 28 | 1 | 27 | 4 | 19 |
| Powdered cake | 1 | 330 | 36 | 1 | 35 | 4 | 19 |
| Strawberry | 1 | 210 | 32 | 1 | 31 | 3 | 8 |
| Strawberry-frosted | 1 | 210 | 30 | 1 | 29 | 3 | 9 |
| Sugar raised | 1 | 170 | 22 | 1 | 21 | 3 | 8 |
| Vanilla kreme-filled | 1 | 170 | 36 | 1 | 35 | 3 | 13 |
| Whole white glazed cake | 1 | 310 | 32 | 1 | 31 | 4 | 19 |
| **Donut-Fancies** | | | | | | | |
| Apple fritter | 1 | 300 | 41 | 1 | 40 | 4 | 14 |

| | Serving Size | Calories (g) | Total Carbs(g) | Fiber (g) | Net Carbs(g) | Protein (g) | Fat (g) |
|---|---|---|---|---|---|---|---|
| Bow tie donut | 1 | 300 | 34 | 1 | 33 | 4 | 17 |
| Chocolate-frosted coffee roll | 1 | 290 | 36 | 1 | 35 | 4 | 15 |
| Chocolate-iced Bismarck | 1 | 340 | 50 | 1 | 49 | 3 | 15 |
| Coffee roll | 1 | 270 | 33 | 1 | 32 | 4 | 14 |
| Éclair | 1 | 270 | 39 | 1 | 38 | 4 | 11 |
| Glazed fritter | 1 | 260 | 31 | 1 | 30 | 4 | 14 |
| Maple-frosted coffee roll | 1 | 290 | 36 | 1 | 35 | 4 | 14 |
| Vanilla-frosted coffee roll | 1 | 290 | 36 | 1 | 35 | 4 | 14 |
| **Donut-Munchkins** | | | | | | | |
| Cinnamon cake | 4 | 275 | 31 | 1 | 30 | 3 | 15 |
| Glazed | 5 | 200 | 27 | 1 | 26 | 3 | 9 |
| Glazed cake | 3 | 280 | 38 | 1 | 37 | 3 | 13 |
| Glazed chocolate cake | 3 | 200 | 26 | 1 | 25 | 2 | 10 |
| Jelly-filled | 5 | 210 | 30 | 1 | 29 | 3 | 9 |
| Lemon-filled | 4 | 170 | 23 | 0 | 23 | 2 | 8 |
| Plain cake | 4 | 270 | 27 | 1 | 26 | 3 | 16 |
| Powdered cake | 4 | 270 | 31 | 1 | 30 | 3 | 14 |
| Sugar raised | 7 | 220 | 26 | 1 | 25 | 4 | 12 |
| **Donut-Sticks** | | | | | | | |
| Cinnamon cake | 1 | 450 | 42 | 1 | 39 | 4 | 30 |
| Glazed cake | 1 | 490 | 51 | 1 | 50 | 4 | 29 |
| Glazed chocolate cake | 1 | 470 | 49 | 2 | 47 | 4 | 29 |
| Jelly | 1 | 530 | 61 | 1 | 60 | 4 | 29 |
| Plain cake | 1 | 420 | 35 | 1 | 34 | 4 | 29 |
| Powdered cake | 1 | 450 | 42 | 1 | 41 | 4 | 29 |
| **Muffins** | | | | | | | |
| Banana walnut | 1 | 545 | 73 | 3 | 70 | 10 | 23 |
| Blueberry | 1 | 490 | 75 | 2 | 73 | 8 | 18 |
| Carrot walnut spice | 1 | 600 | 81 | 3 | 78 | 8 | 27 |
| Chocolate chip | 1 | 590 | 85 | 3 | 82 | 9 | 23 |
| Coffee cake with topping | 1 | 710 | 102 | 2 | 100 | 11 | 29 |
| Corn | 1 | 510 | 81 | 1 | 80 | 9 | 17 |
| Cranberry orange | 1 | 460 | 71 | 3 | 68 | 8 | 16 |
| Honey bran raisin | 1 | 490 | 81 | 5 | 76 | 10 | 14 |
| Reduced fat blueberry | 1 | 450 | 74 | 2 | 72 | 9 | 13 |
| **Other Misc. Items** | | | | | | | |
| Apple pie | 1 svg | 615 | 82 | 4 | 78 | 9 | 28 |
| Apple pie a la mode | 1 svg | 810 | 107 | 4 | 103 | 12 | 38 |
| Biscuit, plain | 1 | 250 | 29 | 1 | 28 | 5 | 13 |

| | Serving Size | Calories (g) | Total Carbs(g) | Fiber (g) | Net Carbs(g) | Protein (g) | Fat (g) |
|---|---|---|---|---|---|---|---|
| Croissant, plain | 1 | 330 | 37 | 0 | 37 | 5 | 18 |
| Scone, maple walnut | 1 | 470 | 62 | 1 | 61 | 6 | 22 |
| Scone, raspberry white choc. | 1 | 450 | 59 | 2 | 57 | 6 | 22 |
| **Sandwiches, Breakfast type** | | | | | | | |
| Bagel w/ egg, bacon, cheese | 1 | 500 | 71 | 2 | 69 | 26 | 13 |
| Bagel w/ egg, ham, cheese | 1 | 500 | 70 | 2 | 68 | 29 | 11 |
| Bagel w/ egg, sausage, cheese | 1 | 675 | 71 | 2 | 69 | 32 | 28 |
| Biscuit w/ egg & cheese | 1 | 360 | 31 | 1 | 30 | 14 | 20 |
| Biscuit w/ sausage, egg, cheese | 1 | 560 | 31 | 1 | 30 | 23 | 38 |
| Croissant w/ egg, ham, cheese | 1 | 470 | 38 | 0 | 38 | 20 | 27 |
| English muffin w/egg, cheese | 1 | 270 | 35 | 1 | 34 | 15 | 8 |
| English muffin w/ egg, bacon & cheese | 1 | 310 | 35 | 1 | 34 | 18 | 11 |
| English muffin w/ egg, ham, & cheese | 1 | 310 | 35 | 1 | 34 | 21 | 10 |
| **Beverages** | | | | | | | |
| Cappuccino | 10 oz | 80 | 7 | 0 | 7 | 4 | 5 |
| Cappuccino with sugar | 10 oz | 130 | 21 | 0 | 21 | 4 | 5 |
| *Coffee* | *10 oz* | *15* | *3* | *0* | *3* | *1* | *0* |
| *Coffee with cream* | *10 oz* | *70* | *3* | *0* | *3* | *1* | *6* |
| Coffee with cream and sugar | 10 oz | 120 | 15 | 0 | 15 | 1 | 6 |
| *Coffee with milk* | *10 oz* | *35* | *4* | *0* | *4* | *2* | *1* |
| Coffee with milk and sugar | 10 oz | 80 | 16 | 0 | 16 | 2 | 1 |
| *Coffee with skim milk* | *10 oz* | *25* | *4* | *0* | *4* | *2* | *0* |
| Coffee w/ skim milk and sugar | 10 oz | 70 | 16 | 0 | 16 | 2 | 0 |
| Coffee with sugar | 10 oz | 60 | 15 | 0 | 15 | 1 | 0 |
| Coffee coolatta with 2% milk | 16 oz | 190 | 41 | 0 | 41 | 4 | 2 |
| Coffee coolatta with cream | 16 oz | 350 | 40 | 0 | 40 | 3 | 22 |

| | Serving Size | Calories (g) | Total Carbs(g) | Fiber (g) | Net Carbs(g) | Protein (g) | Fat (g) |
|---|---|---|---|---|---|---|---|
| Coffee coolatta with milk | 16 oz | 210 | 42 | 0 | 42 | 4 | 4 |
| Coffee coolatta with skim milk | 16 oz | 170 | 41 | 0 | 41 | 4 | 0 |
| Coolatta, lemonade | 16 oz | 240 | 59 | 0 | 59 | 0 | 0 |
| Coolatta, orange mango | 16 oz | 270 | 66 | 2 | 64 | 1 | 0 |
| Coolatta, strawberry fruit | 16 oz | 290 | 72 | 1 | 71 | 0 | 0 |
| Coolatta, vanilla bean | 16 oz | 440 | 70 | 1 | 69 | 1 | 17 |
| Dunkaccino | 10 oz | 230 | 35 | 0 | 35 | 2 | 10 |
| *Espresso* | *2 oz* | *1* | *1* | *0* | *1* | *0* | *0* |
| Espresso with sugar | 2 oz | 30 | 7 | 0 | 7 | 0 | 0 |
| Hot chocolate | 10 oz | 220 | 38 | 2 | 36 | 2 | 8 |
| Latte, plain | 10 oz | 120 | 10 | 0 | 10 | 6 | 6 |
| Latte with sugar | 10 oz | 160 | 22 | 0 | 22 | 6 | 6 |
| Latte w/ Caramel swirl | 10 oz | 230 | 36 | 0 | 36 | 8 | 6 |
| Latte w/ Mocha swirl | 10 oz | 230 | 37 | 1 | 36 | 6 | 7 |
| *Iced coffee* | *16 oz* | *15* | *3* | *0* | *3* | *1* | *0* |
| *Iced coffee with cream* | *16 oz* | *70* | *4* | *0* | *4* | *2* | *6* |
| Iced coffee w/ cream and sugar | 16 oz | 120 | 16 | 0 | 16 | 2 | 6 |
| *Iced coffee with milk* | *16 oz* | *35* | *4* | *0* | *4* | *2* | *1* |
| Iced coffee w/ milk and sugar | 16 oz | 80 | 16 | 0 | 16 | 2 | 1 |
| *Iced coffee with skim milk* | *16 oz* | *25* | *4* | *0* | *4* | *2* | *0* |
| Iced coffee w/skim milk, sugar | 16 oz | 70 | 16 | 0 | 16 | 2 | 0 |
| Iced coffee with sugar | 16 oz | 60 | 15 | 0 | 15 | 1 | 0 |
| Iced latte | 16 oz | 120 | 11 | 0 | 11 | 6 | 7 |
| Iced latte with sugar | 16 oz | 170 | 23 | 0 | 23 | 6 | 7 |
| Iced caramel swirl latte | 16 oz | 240 | 37 | 0 | 37 | 8 | 7 |
| Iced mocha swirl latte | 16 oz | 240 | 38 | 1 | 37 | 7 | 8 |
| Vanilla chai | 10 oz | 230 | 40 | 0 | 40 | 1 | 8 |
| Tea, plain, w/o milk or sugar | | | | | | | |
| *Decaffeinated tea* | *10 oz* | *0* | *1* | *0* | *1* | *0* | *0* |
| *Earl Grey tea* | *10 oz* | *0* | *1* | *0* | *1* | *0* | *0* |
| *English breakfast tea* | *10 oz* | *0* | *1* | *0* | *1* | *0* | *0* |
| *Green tea* | *10 oz* | *0* | *1* | *0* | *1* | *0* | *0* |

| | Serving Size | Calories | Total Carbs(g) | Fiber (g) | Net Carbs(g) | Protein (g) | Fat (g) |
|---|---|---|---|---|---|---|---|
| *Regular tea* | *10 oz* | *0* | *1* | *0* | *1* | *0* | *0* |
| *Regular tea w/ lemon* | *10 oz* | *0* | *1* | *0* | *1* | *0* | *0* |
| *Tea w/ regular milk, no sugar* | *10 oz* | *25* | *2* | *0* | *2* | *1* | *1* |
| Tea w/ regular milk and sugar | 10 oz | 70 | 14 | 0 | 14 | 1 | 1 |
| *Tea w/ skim milk, no sugar* | *10 oz* | *25* | *4* | *0* | *4* | *1* | *Tr* |
| Tea w/ skim milk and sugar | 10 oz | 60 | 14 | 0 | 14 | 1 | Tr |
| **Hardees** | | | | | | | |
| Apple cinnamon raisin biscuit | 1 | 200 | 30 | 2 | 28 | 2 | 8 |
| Bacon & egg biscuit | 1 | 575 | 45 | 2 | 43 | 22 | 33 |
| Bacon, egg & cheese biscuit | 1 | 610 | 45 | 2 | 43 | 24 | 37 |
| Baked beans | 1 svg | 170 | 32 | 4 | 28 | 8 | 1 |
| Big chocolate chip cookie | 1 | 280 | 41 | 2 | 39 | 4 | 12 |
| Big country bacon | 1 svg | 820 | 62 | 2 | 60 | 33 | 49 |
| Big country sausage | 1 svg | 995 | 62 | 2 | 60 | 41 | 66 |
| Big roast beef | 1 | 465 | 35 | 3 | 32 | 26 | 24 |
| Biscuits w/ gravy | 1 svg | 495 | 55 | 3 | 52 | 10 | 28 |
| Cheeseburger | 1 | 310 | 30 | 2 | 28 | 16 | 14 |
| Chicken, breast | 1 piece | 370 | 29 | 2 | 27 | 29 | 15 |
| Chicken, leg | 1 piece | 170 | 15 | 1 | 14 | 13 | 7 |
| Chicken, thigh | 1 piece | 330 | 30 | 2 | 28 | 39 | 15 |
| Chicken, wing | 1 piece | 195 | 23 | 1 | 22 | 10 | 8 |
| Chicken fillet sandwich | 1 | 480 | 54 | 3 | 51 | 26 | 18 |
| Chocolate cone | 1 | 180 | 34 | 1 | 33 | 5 | 3 |
| Chocolate shake | 1 | 375 | 67 | 1 | 66 | 13 | 5 |
| Cole slaw | 1 svg | 240 | 13 | 3 | 10 | 2 | 20 |
| Cool twist cone | 1 | 180 | 34 | 1 | 33 | 4 | 2 |
| Country ham biscuit | 1 | 430 | 45 | 3 | 42 | 15 | 22 |

| | Serving Size | Calories (g) | Total Carbs(g) | Fiber (g) | Net Carbs(g) | Protein (g) | Fat (g) |
|---|---|---|---|---|---|---|---|
| Cravin bacon cheeseburger | 1 | 690 | 38 | 2 | 36 | 30 | 46 |
| Fat free French dressing | 1 svg | 70 | 17 | Tr | 17 | 0 | 0 |
| Fisherman's fillet | 1 | 565 | 54 | 3 | 51 | 26 | 27 |
| French fries, Lg | 1 | 430 | 59 | 4 | 55 | 6 | 18 |
| French fries, med | 1 | 350 | 49 | 3 | 46 | 5 | 15 |
| French fries, sm | 1 | 240 | 33 | 2 | 31 | 4 | 10 |
| Frisco ham sandwich | 1 | 500 | 46 | 3 | 43 | 24 | 25 |
| Frisco sandwich | 1 | 720 | 43 | 3 | 40 | 33 | 46 |
| Garden salad | 1 | 220 | 11 | 3 | 8 | 12 | 13 |
| *Gravy, 1.5 oz* | *1 svg* | *22* | *3* | *Tr* | *3* | *1* | *1* |
| Grilled chicken | 1 | 350 | 38 | 2 | 36 | 25 | 11 |
| Chilled chicken salad | 1 | 150 | 11 | 3 | 8 | 20 | 3 |
| Ham biscuit | 1 | 400 | 47 | 3 | 44 | 9 | 30 |
| Ham, egg, & cheese biscuit | 1 | 540 | 48 | 3 | 45 | 20 | 30 |
| Hamburger | 1 | 270 | 29 | 2 | 27 | 14 | 11 |
| Hot fudge sundae | 1 | 180 | 51 | 1 | 50 | 7 | 6 |
| Hot ham & cheese | 1 | 310 | 34 | 2 | 32 | 16 | 12 |
| Jelly biscuit | 1 | 440 | 57 | 3 | 54 | 6 | 21 |
| Mashed potatoes | 1 svg | 70 | 14 | 3 | 11 | 2 | 1 |
| Mesquite bacon cheeseburger | 1 | 370 | 32 | 2 | 30 | 19 | 18 |
| Mushroom & Swiss burger | 1 | 490 | 39 | 2 | 37 | 28 | 25 |
| Pancakes, 3 per svg | 1 svg | 280 | 56 | 3 | 53 | 8 | 2 |
| Peach cobbler | 1 svg | 310 | 60 | 2 | 58 | 2 | 7 |
| Peach shake | 1 | 390 | 77 | 1 | 76 | 10 | 4 |
| Quarter Lb double cheeseburger | 1 | 470 | 31 | 3 | 28 | 27 | 27 |
| Ranch dressing | 1 svg | 290 | 6 | Tr | 6 | 1 | 29 |
| Regular hash rounds | 1 svg | 230 | 24 | 2 | 22 | 3 | 14 |

| | Serving Size | Calories (g) | Total Carbs(g) | Fiber (g) | Net Carbs(g) | Protein (g) | Fat (g) |
|---|---|---|---|---|---|---|---|
| Regular roast beef | 1 | 320 | 26 | 2 | 24 | 17 | 16 |
| Rise & shine biscuit | 1 | 390 | 44 | 2 | 42 | 6 | 21 |
| Sausage biscuit | 1 | 510 | 44 | 2 | 42 | 14 | 31 |
| Sausage & egg biscuit | 1 | 630 | 45 | 2 | 43 | 23 | 40 |
| *Side salad, w/o dressing* | *1* | *25* | *4* | *2* | *2* | *1* | *Tr* |
| Strawberry shake | 1 | 420 | 83 | 1 | 82 | 11 | 4 |
| Strawberry sundae | 1 | 210 | 43 | 1 | 42 | 5 | 2 |
| The boss | 1 | 570 | 42 | 3 | 39 | 27 | 33 |
| The works burger | 1 | 530 | 41 | 3 | 38 | 25 | 30 |
| Thousand Island dressing | 1 svg | 250 | 9 | Tr | 9 | 1 | 23 |
| Ultimate omelet biscuit | 1 | 570 | 45 | 2 | 43 | 22 | 33 |
| Vanilla cone | 1 | 170 | 34 | 1 | 33 | 4 | 2 |
| Vanilla shake | 1 | 350 | 65 | 1 | 64 | 12 | 5 |
| **Jack-In-The-Box** | | | | | | | |
| Breakfast Jack | 1 | 295 | 30 | 1 | 29 | 18 | 12 |
| Breakfast sandwich, sourdough | 1 | 380 | 31 | 2 | 29 | 21 | 20 |
| Carrot cake | 1 piece | 365 | 58 | 2 | 56 | 3 | 15 |
| Cheeseburger, regular | 1 | 320 | 32 | 2 | 30 | 16 | 15 |
| Cheeseburger, double | 1 | 450 | 35 | 2 | 33 | 24 | 24 |
| Cheeseburger, ultimate | 1 | 1025 | 30 | 3 | 27 | 50 | 79 |
| Cheesecake | 1 piece | 310 | 29 | 1 | 28 | 8 | 18 |
| Chicken pita fajita | 1 | 290 | 29 | 2 | 27 | 24 | 8 |
| Chicken sandwich, regular | 1 | 400 | 38 | 2 | 36 | 20 | 18 |
| Chicken sandwich, Caesar | 1 | 520 | 44 | 2 | 42 | 27 | 26 |
| Chicken sandwich, grilled | 1 | 430 | 36 | 2 | 34 | 29 | 19 |
| Chicken sandwich, spicy | 1 | 560 | 55 | 2 | 53 | 24 | 27 |
| Chicken sandwich, super | 1 | 615 | 48 | 2 | 46 | 25 | 36 |
| Chicken strips, 6 per svg | 1 svg | 450 | 28 | 1 | 27 | 39 | 20 |

|  | Serving Size | Calories (g) | Total Carbs(g) | Fiber (g) | Net Carbs(g) | Protein (g) | Fat (g) |
|---|---|---|---|---|---|---|---|
| Chicken teriyaki | 1 svg | 580 | 115 | 5 | 110 | 28 | 2 |
| Egg roll | 1 piece | 150 | 18 | 1 | 17 | 1 | 8 |
| Egg rolls, 5-piece serving | 5 piece | 745 | 92 | 3 | 89 | 5 | 41 |
| French fries, curly, sm | 1 | 400 | 45 | 5 | 40 | 6 | 23 |
| French fries, jumbo size | 1 | 400 | 51 | 3 | 48 | 5 | 19 |
| French fries, regular size | 1 | 350 | 45 | 3 | 42 | 4 | 17 |
| French fries, sm | 1 | 220 | 28 | 2 | 26 | 3 | 11 |
| French fries, super size | 1 | 590 | 76 | 5 | 71 | 8 | 29 |
| Hamburger | 1 | 280 | 31 | 2 | 29 | 13 | 11 |
| Hash browns | 2 oz | 160 | 14 | 2 | 12 | 1 | 11 |
| Jalapenos, stuffed | 1 svg | 600 | 41 | 2 | 39 | 22 | 39 |
| Jumbo Jack | 1 | 560 | 41 | 2 | 39 | 26 | 32 |
| Jumbo Jack w/ cheese | 1 | 650 | 42 | 2 | 40 | 31 | 40 |
| Onion rings | 1 svg | 380 | 38 | 2 | 36 | 5 | 23 |
| Pancake platter | 1 svg | 400 | 59 | 3 | 56 | 13 | 12 |
| Potato wedges, bacon & cheddar | 1 svg | 795 | 49 | 4 | 45 | 20 | 58 |
| Sausage croissant | 1 | 675 | 39 | 2 | 37 | 21 | 48 |
| Scrambled egg pocket | 1 | 430 | 31 | 1 | 30 | 29 | 21 |
| Shake, | | | | | | | |
| Cappuccino | 1 Lg | 625 | 80 | 1 | 79 | 11 | 28 |
| Chocolate | 1 Lg | 625 | 85 | 1 | 84 | 11 | 27 |
| Strawberry | 1 Lg | 630 | 85 | 1 | 84 | 10 | 28 |
| Vanilla | 1 Lg | 615 | 73 | 0 | 73 | 12 | 30 |
| Supreme croissant | 1 | 570 | 39 | 2 | 37 | 21 | 36 |
| Taco | 1 | 185 | 15 | 2 | 13 | 7 | 11 |
| Taco monster | 1 | 285 | 22 | 3 | 19 | 12 | 17 |
| **Kentucky Fried Chicken** | | | | | | | |
| Barbecue baked beans | 1 svg | 185 | 33 | 6 | 27 | 6 | 3 |
| Biscuit | 1 | 180 | 20 | 2 | 18 | 4 | 10 |
| Breast, extra tasty crispy | 1 | 470 | 25 | 1 | 22 | 31 | 28 |
| Breast, hot & spicy | 1 | 520 | 23 | 1 | 22 | 32 | 34 |

| | Serving Size | Calories (g) | Total Carbs(g) | Fiber (g) | Net Carbs(g) | Protein (g) | Fat (g) |
|---|---|---|---|---|---|---|---|
| Breast, original recipe | 1 | 400 | 16 | 1 | 15 | 29 | 25 |
| *Breast, tender roast* | *1* | *255* | *1* | *Tr* | *1* | *29* | *24* |
| Chunky chicken pot pie | 1 | 775 | 69 | 4 | 65 | 29 | 42 |
| Coleslaw | 5 oz | 180 | 21 | 4 | 17 | 2 | 9 |
| Cornbread | 1 piece | 228 | 18 | 3 | 15 | 27 | 13 |
| Corn on the cob | 1 | 190 | 34 | 4 | 30 | 5 | 3 |
| Crispy strips, 3 pieces/svg | 1 svg | 260 | 10 | 3 | 7 | 20 | 16 |
| Drumstick, original recipe | 1 | 160 | 6 | 1 | 5 | 15 | 9 |
| *Drumstick, tender roast* | *1* | *100* | *1* | *0* | *1* | *13* | *4* |
| *Green beans* | *1 svg* | *45* | *7* | *3* | *4* | *1* | *5* |
| Hot wings, 6 pieces/svg | 1 svg | 470 | 18 | 2 | 16 | 27 | 33 |
| Kentucky nuggets, 6 pieces/svg | 1 svg | 285 | 15 | 1 | 14 | 16 | 18 |
| Macaroni and cheese | med | 180 | 21 | 3 | 18 | 7 | 8 |
| Original recipe chicken sandwich | 1 | 495 | 46 | 3 | 43 | 29 | 22 |
| Potato salad | 1 svg | 230 | 23 | 3 | 20 | 4 | 14 |
| Potato wedges | 1 svg | 280 | 28 | 3 | 25 | 5 | 13 |
| Potatoes, mashed | 1 svg | 120 | 17 | 3 | 14 | 1 | 6 |
| Red beans and rice | 1 svg | 130 | 21 | 3 | 18 | 5 | 3 |
| Thigh, extra tasty crispy or hot | 1 | 370 | 18 | 1 | 16 | 19 | 25 |
| Thigh, original recipe | 1 | 255 | 6 | 1 | 5 | 16 | 18 |
| *Thigh, tender roast* | *1* | *205* | *1* | *0* | *1* | *18* | *12* |
| Value BBQ chicken sandwich | 1 | 255 | 28 | 2 | 26 | 17 | 8 |
| Wing, extra tasty crispy or hot | 1 | 210 | 9 | 1 | 8 | 10 | 15 |
| Wing, original recipe | 1 | 140 | 5 | Tr | 5 | 9 | 10 |
| *Wing, tender roast* | *1* | *121* | *1* | *Tr* | *1* | *12* | *8* |
| **Krispy Kreme Doughnuts** | | | | | | | |
| Apple fritter | 1 | 385 | 46 | Tr | 46 | 4 | 21 |

| | Serving Size | Calories (g) | Total Carbs (g) | Fiber (g) | Net Carbs (g) | Protein (g) | Fat (g) |
|---|---|---|---|---|---|---|---|
| Caramel creme crunch | 1 | 350 | 43 | Tr | 43 | 4 | 19 |
| Chocolate-iced cake | 1 | 270 | 36 | Tr | 36 | 3 | 14 |
| Chocolate-iced cake w/ sprinkles | 1 | 290 | 40 | Tr | 40 | 3 | 14 |
| Chocolate-iced crème filled | 1 | 350 | 39 | Tr | 39 | 3 | 21 |
| Chocolate-iced cruller | 1 | 290 | 37 | Tr | 37 | 2 | 15 |
| Chocolate-iced custard filled | 1 | 300 | 35 | Tr | 35 | 3 | 17 |
| Chocolate-iced glazed | 1 | 250 | 33 | Tr | 33 | 3 | 12 |
| Chocolate-iced glazed, sprinkles | 1 | 200 | 38 | Tr | 38 | 3 | 12 |
| Chocolate malted kreme | 1 | 395 | 49 | Tr | 49 | 4 | 21 |
| Cinnamon apple filled | 1 | 290 | 32 | Tr | 32 | 3 | 16 |
| Cinnamon bun | 1 | 260 | 28 | Tr | 28 | 3 | 16 |
| Cinnamon sugar cake | 1 | 280 | 37 | Tr | 37 | 3 | 14 |
| Cinnamon twist | 1 | 230 | 33 | Tr | 33 | 3 | 9 |
| Coffee & kreme | 1 | 360 | 43 | Tr | 43 | 3 | 20 |
| Dulce de leche | 1 | 295 | 30 | Tr | 30 | 3 | 18 |
| Glazed blueberry cake | 1 | 340 | 42 | Tr | 42 | 3 | 18 |
| Glazed blueberry-filled | 1 | 290 | 35 | Tr | 35 | 3 | 16 |
| Glazed cinnamon | 1 | 210 | 24 | Tr | 24 | 2 | 12 |
| Glazed crème-filled | 1 | 345 | 39 | Tr | 39 | 3 | 20 |
| Glazed cruller | 1 | 240 | 26 | Tr | 26 | 2 | 14 |
| Glazed custard-filled | 1 | 290 | 34 | Tr | 34 | 3 | 16 |
| Glazed devil's food cake | 1 | 340 | 42 | Tr | 42 | 3 | 18 |
| Glazed lemon-filled | 1 | 290 | 34 | Tr | 34 | 3 | 16 |
| Glazed sour cream | 1 | 340 | 42 | Tr | 42 | 3 | 18 |
| Glazed raspberry-filled | 1 | 300 | 39 | Tr | 39 | 3 | 16 |
| Glazed strawberry-filled | 1 | 290 | 35 | Tr | 35 | 3 | 16 |
| Glazed twist | 1 | 210 | 28 | Tr | 28 | 3 | 9 |
| Honey and oat | 1 | 340 | 42 | Tr | 42 | 3 | 18 |

| | Serving Size | Calories (g) | Total Carbs(g) | Fiber (g) | Net Carbs(g) | Protein (g) | Fat (g) |
|---|---|---|---|---|---|---|---|
| Key lime pie | 1 | 330 | 40 | Tr | 40 | 3 | 18 |
| Maple-iced | 1 | 240 | 32 | Tr | 32 | 2 | 12 |
| Maple-iced cake | 1 | 270 | 35 | Tr | 35 | 3 | 13 |
| New York cheesecake | 1 | 330 | 36 | Tr | 36 | 4 | 19 |
| Original glazed | 1 | 200 | 22 | Tr | 22 | 2 | 12 |
| Powdered blueberry-filled | 1 | 290 | 32 | Tr | 32 | 3 | 16 |
| Powdered cake | 1 | 280 | 37 | Tr | 37 | 3 | 14 |
| Powdered crème-filled | 1 | 345 | 36 | Tr | 36 | 3 | 21 |
| Powdered raspberry | 1 | 300 | 36 | Tr | 36 | 3 | 16 |
| Powdered strawberry-filled | 1 | 260 | 26 | Tr | 26 | 3 | 16 |
| Pumpkin spice cake | 1 | 340 | 42 | Tr | 42 | 3 | 18 |
| Sugar coated | 1 | 200 | 21 | Tr | 21 | 2 | 12 |
| Traditional cake | 1 | 230 | 25 | Tr | 25 | 3 | 13 |
| Vanilla-iced cake w/ sprinkles | 1 | 270 | 35 | Tr | 35 | 3 | 13 |
| Vanilla-iced crème-filled | 1 | 345 | 38 | Tr | 38 | 3 | 20 |
| Vanilla-iced custard-filled | 1 | 290 | 33 | Tr | 33 | 3 | 16 |
| Vanilla-iced glazed | 1 | 240 | 32 | Tr | 32 | 2 | 12 |
| Vanilla-iced raspberry-filled | 1 | 355 | 50 | Tr | 50 | 3 | 16 |
| Vanilla-iced raspberry glazed | 1 | 355 | 50 | Tr | 50 | 3 | 16 |
| **Long John Silver's** | | | | | | | |
| Cheesesticks, 3 per svg | 1 svg | 165 | 12 | 1 | 11 | 6 | 9 |
| Chicken, battered plank | 1 | 145 | 9 | 1 | 8 | 8 | 8 |
| Chicken sandwich | 1 | 340 | 40 | 2 | 38 | 13 | 14 |
| Chicken sandwich w/ cheese | 1 | 390 | 40 | 2 | 38 | 16 | 19 |
| Clam chowder | 1 svg | 525 | 52 | 4 | 48 | 24 | 24 |
| Clams, breaded | 1 svg | 250 | 26 | 2 | 24 | 9 | 14 |
| Cole slaw | 4 oz | 170 | 23 | 5 | 18 | 2 | 7 |
| Crabcake | 1 | 150 | 12 | 1 | 11 | 4 | 9 |

| | Serving Size | Calories (g) | Total Carbs(g) | Fiber (g) | Net Carbs(g) | Protein (g) | Fat (g) |
|---|---|---|---|---|---|---|---|
| Fish, battered | 1 piece | 230 | 16 | 2 | 14 | 12 | 13 |
| Fish, battered, junior size | 1 piece | 120 | 8 | 1 | 7 | 5 | 8 |
| Fish, country breaded | 1 piece | 200 | 17 | 2 | 15 | 10 | 10 |
| Fish w/lemon crumb | 2 piece | 240 | 10 | 2 | 8 | 23 | 12 |
| Fish sandwich | 1 | 430 | 46 | 3 | 43 | 16 | 20 |
| Fish sandwich w/ cheese | 1 | 485 | 46 | 3 | 43 | 19 | 25 |
| Fish sandwich, ultimate | 1 | 490 | 46 | 3 | 43 | 19 | 26 |
| French fries, reg size | 1 | 250 | 28 | 2 | 26 | 3 | 15 |
| French fries, Lg size | 1 | 420 | 46 | 4 | 42 | 5 | 24 |
| Grilled chicken salad | 1 | 140 | 20 | 3 | 17 | 10 | 3 |
| Hushpuppies | 2 piece | 120 | 50 | 2 | 48 | 18 | 6 |
| Ocean chef salad | 1 | 128 | 15 | 3 | 12 | 14 | 2 |
| Pie, banana split sundae | 1 svg | 300 | 34 | 2 | 32 | 4 | 17 |
| Pie, chocolate crème | 1 svg | 285 | 29 | 3 | 26 | 4 | 17 |
| Pie, Dutch apple | 1 svg | 290 | 44 | 3 | 41 | 2 | 13 |
| Pie, pecan | 1 svg | 390 | 53 | 3 | 50 | 3 | 19 |
| Pie, strawberries & cream | 1 svg | 280 | 32 | 3 | 29 | 4 | 15 |
| Pineapple crème cheesecake | 1 svg | 310 | 36 | 3 | 33 | 4 | 17 |
| *Shrimp, battered* | *1 piece* | *45* | *3* | *1* | *2* | *2* | *3* |
| Shrimp, battered, popcorn | 1 svg | 325 | 33 | 3 | 30 | 15 | 15 |
| **McDonald's** | | | | | | | |
| Apple bran muffin, lowfat | 1 | 300 | 61 | 3 | 58 | 6 | 3 |
| Apple Danish | 1 | 360 | 51 | 1 | 50 | 5 | 16 |
| Apple pie, baked | 1 | 260 | 34 | 1 | 33 | 3 | 13 |
| Arch deluxe | 1 | 550 | 69 | 4 | 65 | 28 | 31 |
| Arch deluxe with bacon | 1 | 590 | 38 | 4 | 34 | 32 | 34 |
| Bacon, egg & cheese biscuit | 1 | 440 | 33 | 1 | 32 | 17 | 26 |
| Barbecue sauce | 1 svg | 45 | 10 | 0 | 10 | 0 | 0 |
| Big mac | 1 | 560 | 45 | 3 | 42 | 26 | 31 |

| | Serving Size | Calories (g) | Total Carbs(g) | Fiber (g) | Net Carbs(g) | Protein (g) | Fat (g) |
|---|---|---|---|---|---|---|---|
| Biscuit, plain | 1 | 260 | 32 | 1 | 31 | 4 | 13 |
| Breakfast burrito | 1 | 320 | 23 | 1 | 22 | 13 | 20 |
| Caesar salad | 1 | 160 | 7 | 0 | 7 | 2 | 14 |
| Chef salad | 1 | 230 | 8 | 3 | 5 | 21 | 13 |
| Cheese Danish | 1 | 410 | 47 | 0 | 47 | 7 | 22 |
| Cheeseburger | 1 | 320 | 35 | 2 | 33 | 15 | 13 |
| Chicken McNuggets, 4 pieces | 1 svg | 190 | 10 | 0 | 10 | 12 | 11 |
| Chicken McNuggets, 6 pieces | 1 svg | 290 | 15 | 0 | 15 | 18 | 17 |
| Chicken McNuggets, 9 pieces | 1 svg | 430 | 23 | 0 | 23 | 27 | 26 |
| Chocolate chip cookie | 1 | 170 | 22 | 1 | 21 | 2 | 10 |
| Chocolate shake, sm | 1 | 360 | 60 | 1 | 59 | 11 | 9 |
| Cinnamon roll | 1 | 400 | 47 | 2 | 45 | 7 | 20 |
| Crispy chicken deluxe | 1 | 500 | 43 | 3 | 40 | 26 | 25 |
| Croutons | 1 svg | 50 | 7 | 0 | 7 | 2 | 5 |
| Egg McMuffin | 1 | 290 | 27 | 1 | 26 | 17 | 12 |
| English muffin | 1 | 140 | 25 | 1 | 24 | 4 | 2 |
| Fat free herb vinegar dressing | 1 svg | 50 | 11 | 0 | 11 | 1 | 0 |
| Fish fillet sandwich | 1 | 560 | 54 | 4 | 50 | 23 | 28 |
| French fries, Lg | 1 | 450 | 57 | 5 | 52 | 6 | 22 |
| French fries, sm | 1 | 210 | 26 | 2 | 24 | 3 | 10 |
| Garden salad | 1 | 35 | 7 | 2 | 5 | 2 | 0 |
| Grilled chicken deluxe | 1 | 440 | 38 | 3 | 35 | 27 | 20 |
| Grilled chicken salad deluxe | 1 | 120 | 7 | 2 | 5 | 21 | 2 |
| Hamburger | 1 | 260 | 34 | 2 | 32 | 13 | 9 |
| Hash browns | 1 svg | 130 | 53 | 2 | 51 | 9 | 7 |
| Honey dressing | 1 svg | 45 | 12 | 0 | 12 | 0 | 0 |
| *Honey mustard dressing* | *1 svg* | *50* | *3* | *0* | *3* | *0* | *5* |

| | Serving Size | Calories (g) | Total Carbs(g) | Fiber (g) | Net Carbs(g) | Protein (g) | Fat (g) |
|---|---|---|---|---|---|---|---|
| Hot caramel sundae | 1 | 360 | 61 | 0 | 61 | 7 | 10 |
| Hot fudge sundae | 1 | 340 | 52 | 1 | 51 | 8 | 12 |
| Hot mustard | 1 svg | 60 | 7 | 0 | 7 | 1 | 4 |
| Hotcakes, plain | 1 svg | 310 | 53 | 2 | 51 | 9 | 7 |
| Hotcakes w/ syrup & margarine | 1 svg | 580 | 100 | 2 | 98 | 9 | 16 |
| *Mayonnaise, light* | *1 svg* | *40* | *0* | *0* | *0* | *0* | *4* |
| McDonaldland cookie | 1 | 180 | 32 | 1 | 31 | 3 | 5 |
| Quarter pounder | 1 | 420 | 37 | 2 | 35 | 23 | 21 |
| Quarter pounder w/ cheese | 1 | 530 | 38 | 2 | 36 | 28 | 30 |
| Red French reduced cal dressing | 1 svg | 160 | 23 | 0 | 23 | 0 | 8 |
| *Sausage (w/o biscuit)* | *1 svg* | *170* | *0* | *0* | *0* | *6* | *16* |
| Sausage biscuit w/ egg | 1 | 505 | 33 | 1 | 32 | 16 | 35 |
| Sausage McMuffin | 1 | 360 | 26 | 1 | 25 | 13 | 23 |
| Sausage McMuffin w/ egg | 1 | 440 | 27 | 1 | 26 | 19 | 28 |
| *Scrambled eggs, 2 per svg* | *1 svg* | *160* | *1* | *0* | *1* | *13* | *11* |
| Strawberry shake, sm | 1 | 360 | 60 | 0 | 60 | 11 | 9 |
| Strawberry sundae | 1 | 290 | 50 | 0 | 50 | 7 | 7 |
| Sweet & sour sauce | 1 svg | 50 | 11 | 0 | 11 | 0 | 0 |
| Vanilla cone, reduced fat | 1 | 150 | 23 | 0 | 23 | 4 | 5 |
| Vanilla shake, sm | 1 | 360 | 59 | 0 | 59 | 11 | 9 |
| **Panda Express Chinese Food** | | | | | | | |
| Beef dishes | | | | | | | |
|   Beef with broccoli | 6 oz | 150 | 8 | 1 | 7 | 11 | 8 |
|   Beef with string beans | 6 oz | 170 | 11 | 2 | 9 | 12 | 9 |
| Chicken dishes | | | | | | | |
|   Black pepper chicken | 6 oz | 180 | 10 | 2 | 8 | 13 | 10 |

| | Serving Size | Calories (g) | Total Carbs(g) | Fiber (g) | Net Carbs(g) | Protein (g) | Fat (g) |
|---|---|---|---|---|---|---|---|
| Chicken & orange sauce | 6 oz | 480 | 50 | 2 | 48 | 21 | 21 |
| Chicken w/ mushrooms | 6 oz | 130 | 7 | 2 | 5 | 11 | 7 |
| Chicken w/ string beans | 6 oz | 170 | 12 | 3 | 9 | 11 | 8 |
| Hot spicy chicken w/ peanuts | 6 oz | 200 | 17 | 4 | 13 | 18 | 7 |
| Mandarin chicken | 6 oz | 250 | 8 | 2 | 6 | 34 | 9 |
| Potatoes w/ chicken | 6 oz | 220 | 17 | 1 | 16 | 12 | 11 |
| Sweet & sour chicken | 4 oz | 310 | 28 | 2 | 26 | 18 | 14 |
| **Pork dishes** | | | | | | | |
| Barbecue pork | 5 oz | 350 | 13 | Tr | 13 | 32 | 19 |
| Sweet & sour pork | 4 oz | 410 | 17 | 3 | 14 | 19 | 30 |
| **Vegetable dishes** | | | | | | | |
| Mixed vegetables | 6 oz | 70 | 8 | 3 | 5 | 3 | 3 |
| String beans w/fried tofu | 6 oz | 180 | 11 | 3 | 8 | 10 | 11 |
| Vegetable chow mein | 8 oz | 330 | 48 | 4 | 44 | 10 | 11 |
| **Rice** | | | | | | | |
| Fried rice w/vegetables | 8 oz | 390 | 61 | 2 | 59 | 9 | 12 |
| Steamed rice | 8 oz | 330 | 74 | 2 | 72 | 7 | 1 |
| **Appetizers** | | | | | | | |
| Fried shrimp | 6 piece | 260 | 26 | Tr | 26 | 12 | 12 |
| Chicken egg roll | 1 | 190 | 21 | 3 | 18 | 8 | 8 |
| Vegetable spring roll | 1 | 80 | 14 | 1 | 13 | 2 | 3 |
| **Sauces** | | | | | | | |
| ***Hot mustard sauce*** | ***1 svg*** | ***18*** | ***1*** | ***0*** | ***1*** | ***0*** | ***0*** |
| ***Hot sauce*** | ***2 tsp*** | ***10*** | ***2*** | ***0*** | ***2*** | ***0*** | ***1*** |
| Mandarin sauce | 2 oz | 70 | 16 | 0 | 16 | Tr | 0 |
| Sweet & sour sauce | 2 oz | 60 | 15 | 0 | 15 | Tr | 0 |
| ***Soy sauce*** | ***1 Tbsp*** | ***16*** | ***2*** | ***0*** | ***2*** | ***2*** | ***0*** |
| **Papa John's Pizza** | | | | | | | |
| Original crust pizza, Lg | 14-inch | | | | | | |
| Cheese | 1 slice | 290 | 39 | 2 | 37 | 12 | 10 |
| Pepperoni | 1 slice | 345 | 39 | 2 | 37 | 14 | 15 |
| Sausage | 1 slice | 335 | 38 | 2 | 36 | 14 | 14 |
| Sausage, pepperoni & beef | 1 slice | 405 | 39 | 2 | 37 | 18 | 20 |

| | Serving Size | Calories (g) | Total Carbs(g) | Fiber (g) | Net Carbs(g) | Protein (g) | Fat (g) |
|---|---|---|---|---|---|---|---|
| Sausage & pepperoni | 1 slice | 348 | 38 | 2 | 36 | 16 | 15 |
| Vegetable garden fresh pizza | 1 slice | 287 | 40 | 3 | 37 | 12 | 9 |
| Works, the works pizza | 1 slice | 370 | 40 | 3 | 37 | 17 | 16 |
| Specialty pizzas | | | | | | | |
| Alfredo, spinach | 1 slice | 303 | 37 | 2 | 35 | 13 | 12 |
| Alfredo, vegetable & chicken | 1 slice | 310 | 37 | 2 | 35 | 15 | 12 |
| Chicken and bacon BBQ | 1 slice | 370 | 44 | 2 | 42 | 17 | 14 |
| Hawaiian BBQ chicken | 1 slice | 375 | 46 | 2 | 44 | 17 | 14 |
| Thin crust pizza, large | 14-inch | | | | | | |
| Cheese | 1 slice | 240 | 23 | 1 | 22 | 10 | 13 |
| Pepperoni | 1 slice | 295 | 23 | 2 | 21 | 12 | 18 |
| Sausage | 1 slice | 303 | 24 | 2 | 22 | 13 | 18 |
| Sausage, pepperoni & beef | 1 slice | 371 | 24 | 2 | 22 | 17 | 24 |
| Sausage & pepperoni | 1 slice | 298 | 23 | 1 | 22 | 13 | 18 |
| Vegetable garden fresh pizza | 1 slice | 228 | 24 | 2 | 22 | 9 | 11 |
| Works, the works pizza | 1 slice | 315 | 25 | 2 | 23 | 14 | 18 |
| Specialty pizzas | | | | | | | |
| Alfredo, spinach | 1 slice | 251 | 22 | 1 | 21 | 10 | 15 |
| Alfredo, vegetable & chicken | 1 slice | 276 | 22 | 1 | 21 | 14 | 15 |
| Chicken and bacon BBQ | 1 slice | 336 | 30 | 1 | 29 | 15 | 18 |
| Hawaiian BBQ chicken | 1 slice | 324 | 31 | 1 | 30 | 14 | 17 |
| Side items | | | | | | | |
| BBQ dipping sauce | 1 svg | 48 | 10 | 0 | 10 | 0 | 0 |
| Bread sticks | 1 svg | 140 | 26 | 1 | 25 | 4 | 2 |
| *Buffalo hot sauce* | *1 svg* | *25* | *3* | *0* | *3* | *0* | *1* |
| *Cheese sauce* | *1 svg* | *60* | *0* | *0* | *0* | *4* | *5* |
| Cheese sticks | 1 svg | 180 | 20 | 1 | 19 | 8 | 8 |
| Chicken strips | 1 svg | 83 | 5 | Tr | 5 | 6 | 4 |
| Cinnapie | 1 svg | 114 | 14 | 0 | 14 | 1 | 6 |
| *Garlic sauce* | *1 svg* | *235* | *0* | *0* | *0* | *0* | *26* |
| Honey mustard dipping sauce | 1 svg | 190 | 6 | 0 | 6 | 0 | 19 |
| *Pizza sauce* | *1 svg* | *25* | *3* | *2* | *1* | *0* | *2* |
| *Ranch dipping sauce* | *1 svg* | *140* | *2* | *0* | *2* | *1* | *14* |

| | Serving Size | Calories (g) | Total Carbs(g) | Fiber (g) | Net Carbs(g) | Protein (g) | Fat (g) |
|---|---|---|---|---|---|---|---|
| **Pizza Hut** | | | | | | | |
| Apple dessert pizza | 1 slice | 255 | 48 | 2 | 46 | 3 | 5 |
| Bread stick | 1 | 130 | 20 | 1 | 19 | 3 | 4 |
| Bread stick sauce for dipping | 1 svg | 30 | 5 | 0 | 5 | 0 | 1 |
| *Buffalo wings, hot* | *4* | *210* | *4* | *0* | *4* | *22* | *12* |
| *Buffalo wings, mild* | *5* | *200* | *0* | *0* | *0* | *23* | *12* |
| Cavatini pasta | 1 svg | 485 | 66 | 9 | 57 | 21 | 14 |
| Cavatini pasta supreme | 1 svg | 565 | 73 | 10 | 63 | 24 | 19 |
| Cherry dessert pizza | 1 slice | 250 | 47 | 3 | 44 | 3 | 5 |
| Garlic bread | 1 slice | 150 | 16 | 1 | 15 | 3 | 8 |
| Ham and cheese sandwich | 1 | 555 | 57 | 4 | 53 | 33 | 21 |
| Hand tossed pizza | | | | | | | |
|   Beef | 1 slice | 260 | 16 | 2 | 14 | 16 | 9 |
|   Cheese | 1 slice | 235 | 29 | 2 | 27 | 12 | 7 |
|   Ham | 1 slice | 215 | 28 | 2 | 26 | 14 | 5 |
|   Pepperoni | 1 slice | 238 | 28 | 2 | 26 | 13 | 8 |
|   Sausage | 1 slice | 265 | 28 | 2 | 26 | 16 | 11 |
|   Supreme | 1 slice | 284 | 29 | 3 | 26 | 13 | 12 |
| Pan pizza | | | | | | | |
|   Beef | 1 slice | 285 | 28 | 2 | 26 | 14 | 13 |
|   Cheese | 1 slice | 260 | 28 | 2 | 26 | 12 | 11 |
|   Ham | 1 slice | 240 | 28 | 2 | 26 | 11 | 9 |
|   Pepperoni | 1 slice | 265 | 28 | 2 | 26 | 11 | 12 |
|   Supreme | 1 slice | 310 | 28 | 3 | 25 | 15 | 15 |
|   Veggie | 1 slice | 245 | 29 | 3 | 26 | 10 | 10 |
| Spaghetti w/marina sauce | 1 svg | 490 | 91 | 8 | 83 | 18 | 6 |
| Spaghetti w/ meat sauce | 1 svg | 600 | 98 | 9 | 89 | 23 | 13 |
| Spaghetti w/meatballs | 1 svg | 850 | 120 | 10 | 110 | 37 | 24 |
| Stuffed crust pizza | | | | | | | |
|   Beef | 1 slice | 465 | 46 | 3 | 43 | 23 | 22 |
|   Cheese | 1 slice | 445 | 46 | 3 | 43 | 22 | 19 |
|   Ham | 1 slice | 404 | 45 | 3 | 42 | 24 | 22 |
|   Pepperoni | 1 slice | 440 | 45 | 3 | 42 | 21 | 19 |
|   Sausage | 1 slice | 480 | 46 | 3 | 43 | 22 | 23 |
| Supreme sandwich | 1 | 640 | 62 | 4 | 58 | 34 | 28 |

| | Serving Size | Calories (g) | Total Carbs(g) | Fiber (g) | Net Carbs(g) | Protein (g) | Fat (g) |
|---|---|---|---|---|---|---|---|
| Thin & crispy pizza | | | | | | | |
| Beef | 1 slice | 230 | 22 | 1 | 21 | 13 | 11 |
| Cheese | 1 slice | 205 | 22 | 1 | 21 | 10 | 8 |
| Ham | 1 slice | 185 | 21 | 1 | 20 | 9 | 7 |
| Pepperoni | 1 slice | 215 | 21 | 1 | 20 | 9 | 10 |
| Sausage | 1 slice | 235 | 22 | 1 | 21 | 12 | 12 |
| Supreme | 1 slice | 255 | 23 | 1 | 22 | 12 | 13 |
| Veggie | 1 slice | 185 | 24 | 2 | 22 | 8 | 7 |
| **Subway** | | | | | | | |
| Six" subs | | | | | | | |
| BLT on wheat | 1 | 325 | 44 | 3 | 41 | 14 | 10 |
| BLT on white | 1 | 310 | 38 | 3 | 35 | 14 | 10 |
| Classic Italian | | | | | | | |
| BMT wheat | 1 | 460 | 45 | 3 | 42 | 21 | 22 |
| Classic Italian | | | | | | | |
| BMT white | 1 | 445 | 39 | 3 | 36 | 21 | 21 |
| Cold cut trio on wheat | 1 | 380 | 46 | 3 | 43 | 20 | 13 |
| Cold cut trio on white | 1 | 360 | 39 | 3 | 36 | 19 | 13 |
| Ham on wheat | 1 | 300 | 45 | 3 | 42 | 19 | 5 |
| Ham on white | 1 | 287 | 39 | 3 | 36 | 18 | 5 |
| Meatball on wheat | 1 | 420 | 51 | 3 | 48 | 19 | 16 |
| Meatball on white | 1 | 405 | 44 | 3 | 41 | 18 | 16 |
| Pizza sub on wheat | 1 | 465 | 48 | 3 | 45 | 19 | 22 |
| Pizza sub on white | 1 | 448 | 41 | 3 | 38 | 19 | 22 |
| Roast beef on wheat | 1 | 305 | 45 | 3 | 42 | 20 | 5 |
| Roast beef on white | 1 | 288 | 39 | 3 | 36 | 19 | 5 |
| Roasted chicken breast on wheat | 1 | 348 | 47 | 3 | 44 | 27 | 6 |
| Roasted chicken breast on white | 1 | 332 | 41 | 3 | 38 | 26 | 6 |
| Spicy Italian on wheat | 1 | 482 | 44 | 3 | 41 | 21 | 25 |
| Spice Italian on white | 1 | 465 | 38 | 3 | 35 | 20 | 24 |
| Steak & cheese on wheat | 1 | 395 | 47 | 3 | 44 | 30 | 10 |
| Steak & cheese on white | 1 | 383 | 41 | 3 | 38 | 29 | 10 |
| Subway club on wheat | 1 | 310 | 46 | 3 | 43 | 21 | 5 |
| Subway club on white | 1 | 295 | 40 | 3 | 37 | 21 | 5 |
| Subway melt on wheat | 1 | 382 | 46 | 3 | 43 | 23 | 12 |
| Subway melt on white | 1 | 366 | 40 | 3 | 37 | 22 | 12 |

| | Serving Size | Calories (g) | Total Carbs(g) | Fiber (g) | Net Carbs(g) | Protein (g) | Fat (g) |
|---|---|---|---|---|---|---|---|
| Subway seafood & crab on wheat | 1 | 430 | 44 | 3 | 41 | 20 | 19 |
| Subway seafood & crab on white | 1 | 415 | 38 | 3 | 35 | 19 | 19 |
| Tuna on wheat | 1 | 542 | 44 | 3 | 41 | 19 | 32 |
| Tuna on white | 1 | 527 | 38 | 3 | 35 | 18 | 32 |
| Turkey breast & ham on wheat | 1 | 280 | 39 | 3 | 36 | 18 | 5 |
| Turkey breast & ham on white | 1 | 295 | 46 | 3 | 43 | 18 | 5 |
| Turkey on wheat | 1 | 289 | 46 | 3 | 43 | 18 | 4 |
| Turkey on white | 1 | 273 | 40 | 3 | 37 | 17 | 4 |
| Veggie delite on wheat | 1 | 235 | 34 | 3 | 31 | 9 | 3 |
| Veggie delite on white | 1 | 220 | 38 | 3 | 35 | 9 | 3 |
| Taco subs | | | | | | | |
| Chicken taco sub on wheat | 1 | 436 | 49 | 4 | 45 | 25 | 16 |
| Chicken taco sub on white | 1 | 421 | 43 | 3 | 40 | 24 | 16 |
| Beverages | | | | | | | |
| Berry lishus drink | sm | 113 | 28 | 1 | 27 | 0 | 0 |
| Peach pizazz drink | sm | 103 | 26 | 1 | 25 | 0 | 0 |
| Pineapple delight drink | sm | 133 | 33 | 1 | 32 | 1 | 0 |
| Sunrise refresher drink | sm | 119 | 29 | 1 | 28 | 1 | 0 |
| Cookies | | | | | | | |
| Brazil nut & chocolate chip | 1 | 230 | 27 | 1 | 26 | 3 | 12 |
| Chocolate chip cookie | 1 | 210 | 29 | 1 | 28 | 2 | 10 |
| Chocolate chip, M&M cookie | 1 | 210 | 29 | 1 | 28 | 2 | 10 |
| Chocolate chunk cookie | 1 | 210 | 29 | 1 | 28 | 2 | 10 |
| Oatmeal raisin cookie | 1 | 205 | 29 | 1 | 28 | 3 | 8 |
| Peanut butter cookie | 1 | 220 | 26 | 1 | 25 | 3 | 12 |
| Sugar cookie | 1 | 230 | 28 | 0 | 28 | 2 | 12 |
| White chip macadamia nut | 1 | 235 | 28 | 0 | 28 | 2 | 12 |
| **Taco Bell** | | | | | | | |
| Bacon cheeseburger | 1 | 565 | 43 | 4 | 39 | 29 | 30 |
| Bean burrito | 1 | 378 | 55 | 12 | 43 | 13 | 12 |

| | Serving Size | Calories (g) | Total Carbs(g) | Fiber (g) | Net Carbs(g) | Protein (g) | Fat (g) |
|---|---|---|---|---|---|---|---|
| Big beef meximelt | 1 | 300 | 21 | 2 | 19 | 16 | 16 |
| Big beef nachos supreme | 1 | 435 | 43 | 9 | 34 | 12 | 24 |
| Big beef supreme | 1 | 518 | 52 | 9 | 43 | 26 | 23 |
| Breakfast cheese quesadilla | 1 | 390 | 32 | 1 | 31 | 0 | 22 |
| Breakfast quesadilla w/ bacon | 1 | 465 | 33 | 1 | 32 | 1 | 28 |
| Breakfast quesadilla w/ sausage | 1 | 440 | 33 | 1 | 32 | 0 | 26 |
| Burrito supreme | 1 | 440 | 50 | 8 | 42 | 19 | 18 |
| *Cheddar cheese* | *1 svg* | *30* | *0* | *0* | *0* | *2* | *2* |
| Cheese quesadilla | 1 | 370 | 32 | 1 | 31 | 16 | 20 |
| Chicken club | 1 | 540 | 43 | 4 | 39 | 22 | 31 |
| Chicken fajita | 1 | 460 | 49 | 3 | 46 | 18 | 21 |
| Chicken fajita supreme | 1 | 500 | 51 | 3 | 48 | 19 | 25 |
| Chicken quesadilla | 1 | 420 | 33 | 1 | 32 | 24 | 22 |
| Chili w/ cheese | 1 svg | 330 | 43 | 4 | 39 | 22 | 13 |
| Cinnamon twists | 1 svg | 140 | 19 | 0 | 19 | 1 | 6 |
| Country burrito | 1 | 270 | 26 | 1 | 25 | 1 | 14 |
| Double bacon & egg burrito | 1 | 480 | 39 | 2 | 37 | 2 | 27 |
| Double decker supreme | 1 | 390 | 39 | 8 | 31 | 16 | 18 |
| Double decker taco | 1 | 340 | 37 | 8 | 29 | 16 | 15 |
| Fiesta burrito | 1 | 280 | 25 | 1 | 24 | 1 | 16 |
| Grande burrito | 1 | 420 | 43 | 2 | 41 | 2 | 22 |
| *Green sauce* | *1 svg* | *5* | *1* | *0* | *1* | *0* | *0* |
| *Guacamole* | *1 svg* | *35* | *2* | *1* | *1* | *0* | *3* |
| *Hot taco sauce* | *1 svg* | *0* | *0* | *0* | *0* | *0* | *0* |
| Kid's soft taco roll-up | 1 | 290 | 20 | 2 | 18 | 16 | 16 |
| Light chicken | 1 | 310 | 41 | 3 | 38 | 18 | 8 |
| Light chicken soft taco | 1 | 180 | 21 | 2 | 19 | 13 | 5 |
| Light chicken supreme | 1 | 430 | 52 | 3 | 49 | 25 | 13 |

| | Serving Size | Calories (g) | Total Carbs(g) | Fiber (g) | Net Carbs(g) | Protein (g) | Fat (g) |
|---|---|---|---|---|---|---|---|
| Light kid's chicken soft taco | 1 | 180 | 20 | 1 | 19 | 13 | 5 |
| Mexican pizza | 1 | 570 | 41 | 6 | 35 | 21 | 36 |
| Mexican rice | 1 svg | 190 | 20 | 0 | 20 | 6 | 10 |
| *Mild taco sauce* | *1 svg* | *0* | *0* | *0* | *0* | *0* | *0* |
| Nacho cheese sauce | 1 svg | 120 | 5 | 0 | 5 | 2 | 10 |
| Nachos | 1 | 315 | 34 | 3 | 31 | 2 | 18 |
| Nachos belle grande | 1 | 740 | 83 | 17 | 66 | 16 | 39 |
| *Pepper jack cheese* | *1 svg* | *25* | *1* | *0* | *1* | *0* | *2* |
| *Picante sauce* | *1 svg* | *0* | *1* | *0* | *1* | *0* | *0* |
| Pinto & cheese | 1 | 195 | 18 | 10 | 8 | 9 | 8 |
| *Red sauce* | *1 svg* | *10* | *2* | *0* | *2* | *0* | *0* |
| Salsa | 1 svg | 25 | 5 | 0 | 5 | 1 | 0 |
| Seven layer burrito | 1 | 540 | 65 | 14 | 51 | 16 | 24 |
| Soft taco | 1 | 210 | 20 | 2 | 18 | 12 | 10 |
| Soft taco, BLT | 1 | 340 | 22 | 2 | 20 | 11 | 23 |
| Soft taco, steak | 1 | 510 | 50 | 3 | 47 | 21 | 25 |
| Steak fajita | 1 | 465 | 49 | 3 | 46 | 18 | 21 |
| Taco, hard shell | 1 | 200 | 18 | 1 | 17 | 14 | 7 |
| Taco salad | 1 | 170 | 11 | 1 | 10 | 10 | 10 |
| Taco salad with salsa w/o shell | 1 | 420 | 29 | 13 | 16 | 26 | 21 |
| Taco supreme | 1 | 260 | 22 | 2 | 20 | 13 | 14 |
| Tostada | 1 | 305 | 31 | 11 | 20 | 11 | 14 |
| Veggie fajita | 1 | 420 | 51 | 3 | 48 | 11 | 19 |
| Veggie fajita supreme | 1 | 465 | 53 | 3 | 50 | 11 | 23 |
| **Wendy's** | | | | | | | |
| Baked potato | | | | | | | |
| w/ bacon & cheese | 1 | 535 | 78 | 3 | 75 | 17 | 18 |
| w/ broccoli, cheese | 1 | 470 | 80 | 3 | 77 | 9 | 14 |
| w/ cheese | 1 | 570 | 78 | 3 | 75 | 14 | 23 |
| w/ chili & cheese | 1 | 625 | 83 | 3 | 80 | 20 | 24 |

| | Serving Size | Calories (g) | Total Carbs(g) | Fiber (g) | Net Carbs(g) | Protein (g) | Fat (g) |
|---|---|---|---|---|---|---|---|
| Baked potato w/ sour cream, chive | 1 | 370 | 73 | 3 | 70 | 7 | 5 |
| Big bacon classic hamburger | 1 | 640 | 44 | 2 | 42 | 37 | 36 |
| Breaded chicken fillet | 1 | 220 | 11 | 2 | 9 | 21 | 10 |
| Breaded chicken sandwich | 1 | 450 | 43 | 2 | 41 | 16 | 20 |
| *Caesar salad* | *1* | *110* | *6* | *2* | *4* | *9* | *6* |
| Cheeseburger kids' meal | 1 | 310 | 33 | 2 | 31 | 187 | 13 |
| Chicken Caesar pita | 1 | 485 | 48 | 2 | 46 | 30 | 19 |
| Chicken club sandwich | 1 | 520 | 44 | 3 | 41 | 30 | 25 |
| Chicken nuggets, 5 per svg | 1 svg | 190 | 9 | 2 | 7 | 9 | 13 |
| Chili (Lg) | 1 svg | 310 | 32 | 1 | 31 | 23 | 10 |
| Chili (sm) | 1 svg | 210 | 21 | 1 | 20 | 15 | 7 |
| Chocolate chip cookie | 1 | 270 | 38 | 1 | 37 | 4 | 11 |
| Classic Greek pita | 1 | 440 | 50 | 1 | 49 | 16 | 20 |
| Classic hamburger, single | 1 | 360 | 45 | 1 | 44 | 24 | 16 |
| Classic hamburger w/ everything | 1 | 420 | 31 | 2 | 29 | 25 | 20 |
| *Coleslaw* | *1 svg* | *45* | *5* | *1* | *4* | *0* | *3* |
| French fries (biggie) | 1 | 470 | 61 | 4 | 57 | 7 | 23 |
| French fries (sm) | 1 | 270 | 35 | 2 | 33 | 4 | 13 |
| French fries (super) | 1 | 570 | 73 | 5 | 68 | 8 | 27 |
| Frosty (Lg) | 1 | 570 | 95 | 5 | 90 | 15 | 17 |
| Frosty (med) | 1 | 460 | 76 | 4 | 72 | 12 | 13 |
| Frosty (sm) | 1 | 340 | 57 | 3 | 54 | 9 | 10 |
| Garden ranch chicken pita | 1 | 480 | 51 | 2 | 49 | 27 | 18 |
| Garden veggie pita | 1 | 400 | 52 | 3 | 49 | 11 | 17 |
| *Grilled chicken fillet, w/o bun* | *1* | *100* | *0* | *0* | *0* | *19* | *3* |
| Grilled chicken salad | 1 | 190 | 10 | 2 | 8 | 22 | 8 |
| Grilled chicken sandwich | 1 | 290 | 35 | 2 | 33 | 24 | 7 |
| Hamburger kids' meal | 1 | 270 | 33 | 2 | 31 | 15 | 9 |

| | Serving Size | Calories (g) | Total Carbs(g) | Fiber (g) | Net Carbs(g) | Protein (g) | Fat (g) |
|---|---|---|---|---|---|---|---|
| Junior bacon cheeseburger | 1 | 445 | 33 | 2 | 31 | 22 | 25 |
| Junior cheeseburger | 1 | 320 | 34 | 2 | 32 | 18 | 13 |
| Junior cheeseburger deluxe | 1 | 360 | 36 | 2 | 34 | 18 | 17 |
| Junior hamburger | 1 | 270 | 34 | 2 | 32 | 15 | 9 |
| Kaiser bun | 1 | 190 | 36 | 2 | 34 | 6 | 3 |
| Sandwich bun | 1 | 160 | 29 | 2 | 27 | 5 | 3 |
| Spicy chicken sandwich | 1 | 415 | 43 | 3 | 40 | 28 | 15 |
| Strawberry banana dessert | 1 | 30 | 8 | 1 | 7 | Tr | 0 |
| Taco salad | 1 | 375 | 28 | 1 | 27 | 26 | 19 |
| **White Castle** | | | | | | | |
| Breakfast sandwich, regular | 1 | 335 | 17 | 1 | 16 | 14 | 25 |
| Cheeseburger | 1 | 235 | 11 | 1 | 10 | 7 | 14 |
| Cheeseburger w/ bacon | 1 | 200 | 12 | 1 | 11 | 10 | 13 |
| Cheeseburger, double | 1 | 285 | 12 | 1 | 11 | 14 | 18 |
| Cheesesticks, 5 per svg | 1 svg | 490 | 32 | 1 | 31 | 25 | 28 |
| Chicken rings, 6 per svg | 1 svg | 310 | 17 | 2 | 15 | 16 | 21 |
| Chicken ring sandwich | 1 | 170 | 15 | 2 | 13 | 5 | 7 |
| Chocolate shake | 14 oz | 220 | 32 | 1 | 31 | 8 | 7 |
| Fish sandwich | 1 | 160 | 18 | 1 | 17 | 8 | 6 |
| French fries, sm | 1 | 115 | 15 | 1 | 14 | 1 | 6 |
| Hamburger | 1 | 135 | 11 | 1 | 10 | 6 | 7 |
| Hamburger, double | 1 | 235 | 16 | 1 | 15 | 11 | 14 |
| Onion rings, 8 per svg | 1 svg | 455 | 45 | 1 | 44 | 12 | 25 |
| Vanilla shake | 14 oz | 228 | 35 | 0 | 35 | 8 | 7 |